Healing and Holiness

Healing and Holiness

Sondra Ray

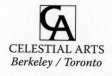

CELESTIAL ARTS
Berkeley / Toronto

Dedication

I give all my credit to my masters Babaji and Ammachi.

I dedicate this book to Sharda, my best friend and spiritual sister; who has expanded my creativity and supported all my projects, helped me perfect and heal myself, made me more enlightened, supported me in every crisis, and enabled me to express my divinity with her in a manner in which we serve together in bliss and peace.

And to Ethel, my mother, who allowed me to be different, taught me very high thoughts, and grounded me in strength and who even now assists Sharda and me from the other side in our current work.

Celestial Arts
P.O. Box 7123
Berkeley, California 94707
www.tenspeed.com

Distributed in Australia by Simon and Schuster Australia, in Canada by Ten Speed Press Canada, in New Zealand by Southern Publishers Group, in South Africa by Real Books, in Southeast Asia by Berkeley Books, and in the United Kingdom and Europe by Airlift Book Company.

Library of Congress Cataloging-in-Publication Data
Ray, Sondra.
    Healing and holiness/ by Sondra Ray.
       p.   cm.
    Includes bibliographical references.
    ISBN 1-58761-161-9
    1. Self-actualization (Psychology) 2. Spiritual healing. I. Title.

BF637.S4 R42 2002
234'.131—dc21   20002074070

Cover design by Leslie Waltzer
Text design by Jeff Brandenburg/ImageComp
World-Healer Mandala © 2001 Bonnie Bell and David Todd (www.gaiastarworld.com)
Astronomical photographs supplied by David Malin Images
Back cover author photo by Mara

First printing, 2002
Printed in Canada

1 2 3 4 5 6 7 8 9 10 — 06 05 04 03 02

Contents

PART I

Background

Foreword

My master Babaji always used to say to those of us who had come to India, "I could heal you all instantly, but what would you learn?"

So then we had to learn to work out our problems by ourselves. Of course, we always learned much more quickly with Babaji's support. And he often took pity on us and took on some of our karma to lighten our loads. With and without Babaji's guidance, I have certainly had my share of "learning experiences" that I do not care to repeat. Somehow I have been good at helping others heal themselves, but I have not been such a good healer for myself. In fact, although I have been a healer since day one, I was hesitant to write a book on this subject until I felt myself reasonably well healed.

Even though a miracle occurred at my birth—my grandfather was instantly healed at the sight of me—I always felt I had failed because of my father's death. My father was sick during most of my life, and I often took care of him, starting at only three years old. When I was six, I told him exactly how to heal himself! That was too much of a shock for my family, and they reprimanded me for being so presumptuous. Watching him slowly dying day by day was devastating.

My preoccupation with healing started with my childhood conditioning. I became a nurse to understand why people get sick and die, but I did not find the answers for which I intuitively looked in Western medicine. I wanted to see permanent healing, not the same symptoms recurring in patients who returned to hospitals again and again. I desperately wanted to know how to prevent disease and death.

I was taught that the Bible said, "In God, all things are possible." I took this promise literally and believed that as a child of God, therefore, I deserved to know how to be permanently healed and how to live forever! If all things were possible, surely this included Physical Immortality. After all, Immortals were mentioned in the Bible.

My father was in and out of hospitals all of my childhood. I have written about this before. What disturbed me most about his chronic illness was that "modern" medicine and religion failed him. He died—and I did not understand why. Later, modern medicine and religion failed for me as well. And they failed my sister who died of melanoma. I ended up divorced, with my hair falling out and in continuous physical pain that lasted twelve to fourteen years. Nobody in modern medicine could help me, so I began searching for other answers.

Finally I was able to begin a real journey of self-healing with alternative methods. But I have had to learn a lot and basically recondition myself about what *healing* really means. This book is an attempt to share with others what I have learned thus far in my healing journey, but it is definitely not my last word on this subject. I am still improving!

I used to blame modern medicine and religion. But now I know that "*truth cannot deal with errors that we want.*" That statement from *A Course in Miracles* is deep enough for a whole chapter alone. Why we want to keep our errors rather than to be healed is a very deep subject. We may think we want to be healed, but our unconscious sabotage patterns are stronger than we realize. Our challenge is to understand how the unconscious mind works and learn how to change it. I wrote this book for those who really want to be permanently healed and for those who want to help others discover how to do the same.

I wondered, after writing fourteen books, "How could any book block me as much as this one? How could any book I would write cause so much commotion? What *was* it about this book?" It seemed to have a power of its own—it kept disappearing.

Perhaps it was because I had to face myself even more than when I wrote my other books. Perhaps it was because I had to review parts of my life that I could hardly remember. Perhaps it was because I did not feel healed enough to complete it, even though I had healed myself of so many ailments. More problems always seemed to come up, and I wanted to be in integrity with what I was writing and really live my words. I guess I felt I was not healed and I was not whole until every single thing in my life worked perfectly. Maybe I could finally heal my body, but what about my other situations? Maybe my relationships with men were finally working, but what about the money case? I could not seem to save money. Then one day I realized that if I waited until everything in my life worked perfectly, I would never get this book out. Maybe Leonard Orr was right when he said that it takes hundreds of years to get your case cracked.

So on a Palm Sunday in Spain, I began this book again. It is the only book of fifteen that I had to completely rewrite twice! I had started it in Spain about four years earlier in the winter. I remember it was cold and I was fed up being without central heating in Old Madrid. Also, it was soon after my sister had died and I was very sad. Her religion had not healed her, and she was not interested in alternative techniques. What right did I have to think that I could be permanently healed? It brought back all the memories and emotions of my father's long illness and death. The thought of all that death was overwhelming.

The manuscript got lost. My publishers lost their copy too. Later I found out they were very sad, for they had lost an endeared editor to AIDS—the one who used to edit my books! We were all bereaved, and none of us could handle a book on *permanent healing* when people we loved were dying.

And yet, that was precisely why I wanted to write this book. Wasn't there any hope? I was holding Jesus to the promise in the Bible that "all things are possible." My higher self was absolutely convinced that it was possible to live in the body free of sickness and pain. I was convinced that we could even stop the aging process if, in fact, "all things are possible." But my lower self had obviously not cleared all the doubts that stood in the way of my faith, because I still could not get this book back. In time, though, it came back. I don't even remember now how I found it, because I had even lost the computer disks. I remembered then that this had happened to me once before: Ideal Birth had disappeared twice. When things are not right, they will not happen or they are just gone, and they come back when I am ready. My gurus protect me this way. I tried to write this book again in Japan at one point and was really proud that I had started over. I wrote for three days solid on everything I knew about healing. It seemed very comprehensive, and I liked my writing style. But, one day—blip! It all disappeared again! The book disappeared from the computer just like that! A blip like that was always my worst fear about computers. The hard drive had failed, and I did not have the backup disk in. I could not understand what was happening. Maybe I had to live out my worst fears.

Trying to find a computer expert who spoke English in Japan was not easy. The girls I lived with eventually found someone, and he checked my computer forward and backward. He phoned me the next day and could only say he was sorry. The second manuscript, the second attempt at this book, was gone! I admit that I broke down and cried. I had to go through a breathwork session right then and there.

Thankfully, two of my staff, Veronica and Debbi, were there to do breathwork on me. I had to process out more loss. There had been so much loss in my life; so many people dying in my hometown, all the funerals I had to witness, the deaths of my father and my sister, and the loss of my husband. Could I ever be healed of loss?

So, on that Palm Sunday in Spain, I started this book for the third time. I really felt I could push through it. It was spring in Spain, and a man I cared for was coming to spend Easter with me. I was also with Adolfo, and he was a real balance to my energy. And he was with a beautiful woman, a flamenco dancer whom I really liked. If I was born to be a writer, I better get on with it—no matter what.

I have, more or less, tried to experience everything possible in the way of alternative healing. My life has been a great transition away from the addiction to Western medicine. It has also been a great learning period. Every one of those people, with various healing techniques, taught me something new about healing. I have always had a special affinity for healers. I love them as my dearest colleagues, for they quietly work hard in all parts of the world. I have been so blessed to find and meet them, to experience their healing energies, and to just hang out with them. Many of them go unacknowledged for their important spiritual service to humanity, and I want to acknowledge all of them now.

Healing Myself

I could have healed myself more quickly had I known at the times of my "illnesses" all the information that is in this book, especially what I have recently discovered about prayer techniques. You could say that I traveled the "low road" of trial, error, and struggle. This chapter is about that "low road" when I was still addicted to the Western medical models. Remember, I became a nurse and was brainwashed by the conventional system. I was afraid to let go of that system. I thought I needed doctors to survive, and it was that dependence that kept me in weakness and helplessness. As you will see, even after I began to give up those Western methods of healing and to explore alternative methods, I was still addicted to struggle. I made my healing process more difficult than necessary, and I wasted a lot of time worrying I would never get over some of those symptoms. My constant worry considerably slowed down the healing process.

When I finally became disenchanted with my own medical profession, I left it to study spiritual healing. However, even after I left, I was not really free; I was just rebelling. I became arrogant and canceled all my medical insurance. I went without insurance for ten full years to prove that I would never need a doctor again. But my attitude was not right, and eventually my arrogance caught up with me. I had a very humbling experience that forced me to go back and forgive "modern" Western medicine for not healing my father. It took me over a decade to wean myself from the system. I practiced spiritual self-healing as much as possible, but I still sought out medical doctors on a couple of occasions. Realizing that totally mastering self-healing would be a long process, I tried to be patient with myself.

Although this book is about how to heal spiritually without the addiction to modern medicine, there may be times when one's fear of giving up traditional methods is too great to overcome. In those cases, you might need to go to a doctor. But remember not to limit yourself to traditional methods alone. Try other techniques of healing. Before running to a doctor, you may want to try some of the techniques discussed in this book. The goal, then, is self-healing. Ultimately, the prevention of the disease is the real goal.

I would like to honor all those doctors who have taken my workshops and classes in search of alternative spiritual healing. Bless you!

What follows is a record of my physical illnesses and what I have learned from those experiences. I am not proud of all the illnesses and negative physical conditions I have manifested over the years, and I wish that learning had been easier. Perhaps the sharing of my healing journey will help others come through their own physical and spiritual healing much faster. But first, let me tell you about my cats!

The Cat Ashram

As a child, I was very lucky, because my cats always healed me. Believe it or not, I had forty cats at one time! (Of course, my dad never let them in the house. There were just too many of them.) I guess I was too busy taking care of all my cats to get sick.

The temptation to get sick was always very strong in our house, though, as well as in our small Iowa town, with a population of just three hundred. It seemed that people were dying right and left. The worst part of it was that all of us children were required to march to the cemetery every time someone died. I took all those deaths very seriously, because everyone in my town was my "family" in one sense or another.

Then, too, there was my father, whom I absolutely adored. He was sick most of the time, and in and out of hospitals. I loved my father and wanted to be just like him, but I did not want to be sick. So it was a tricky relationship for me.

When I was twelve, my dad apparently had rheumatic fever. Later he died of rheumatic heart disease. When he was in the hospital in neighboring Mason City, Iowa, the nuns never let me in to see him because I was not "old enough." He was always there for a long time, so I used to sneak up the fire escape, crawl through the window, and sit with him on the hospital bed. We usually had just a few minutes together before the nuns discovered me and threw me out.

My dad used to say to the nuns, "You leave her alone." But they never listened and threw me out just the same. He always got better when he saw me. Why is it that the medical profession didn't realize that children can be healers for their parents?

Also when I was twelve, I developed all the same symptoms of rheumatic fever that my father had. I got very sick. The doctors could not find any spirochetes or anything else abnormal in my blood. They told my mother that I had a "pseudo" case—my illness just wasn't real.

"Wow!" I said. "Let me out of here so I can take care of my cats!" I think that experience was the beginning of my body taking on *many* illnesses to make me learn about healing.

My cats always waited for me on my grandparents' porch. I spent a lot of time at their house next door because there was a lot less illness in their home. Whenever my dad visited over there with me, my cats would not budge until I came out and he would have to kick his way through them. They followed me everywhere except when I rode my bike to town.

We had huge yards, many barns, and chicken houses. That was great for the cats and all their litters. Different mother cats had different litters here and there, and somehow, I was in charge of them all—at least I thought so. My cats kept me going. If I felt bad, I could talk to my cats. They sat on the lawn and patiently listened to me while I gave them long lectures and shared all my feelings. They made me feel better and actually healed me. (It was perfect practice for being a public speaker later on. They never interrupted me, walked out, or looked bored!) I always felt better after these sessions, and as a child, I was rarely sick except for that one false alarm. I simply did not have time to think about getting sick.

At night, when my dad and grandpa walked out to the pasture to milk the cows, they deliberately clanged the milk pails together, and all the cats came running. It was like a big parade! My dad and grandpa played a game with my cats, aiming the cow's teat, full of milk, at a certain cat's mouth. (I always wondered which one would be "chosen.") The cats liked this game and went along with it wholeheartedly, and I learned to milk the cows the same way.

Every hay season my grandpa came over to our house, opened the door, and yelled, "Sondie, there is a new litter of kittens in the hay barn." Then he shut the door and headed for the hayloft. I ran after him as fast as I could and climbed up the wooden slats to the loft. So many hay bales were always piled up in so many ways that it took me a long time to find the new litter. It was exciting beyond belief, especially when I finally found them.

Sometimes I felt that certain cats were not very good mothers, and in such cases, when they ignored their young, I had wet nurses on the side. Blackie was the best surrogate mother, and she was always willing to nurse kittens that I felt were ignored. When my Blackie died, old and blind, I was devastated. I held a major funeral for her, and all the cats had to attend. After all, that was the way it was done in our town!

I remember a picture of myself taken on one of my birthdays. My mom had put my angel cake on the sidewalk, and the cats came and licked off the frosting. I had long curls with green bows on the tops, and the picture reminds me of how I shared everything with my cats. One day my grandpa gave me a big tent, and my dad built a wooden floor for it and put in electricity. I had a bed in there, and I was in heaven because I could sleep with my cats! I was out there even during heavy rainstorms. Blackie always had top priority and got to sleep by my face. She was, after all, the best mother and "healer" of my cat family.

My cats were my gurus and my healers when I was young. They took care of me and I took care of them. Even after I went off to college, my cats waited for me to come home.

The most amazing thing happened to me when I got older and became a successful writer. My publishers produced a book called *Why Cats Paint.* Phil, the owner of the publishing company, had so much fun doing that book—almost as much fun as I had as a kid with my cats. He even had a display in the gallery below the publishing house of real, live cats painting while people watched. Apparently, certain cats really do love to paint. (Maybe some of my cats followed me in spirit to the publishing company to write their own books!)

When I went to college and left my cat ashram, all the trouble with my "physical conditions" began. For one thing, my father had just died. He died the night before I was to graduate with honors from high school. I was salutatorian and missed being valedictorian by one point. The salutatorian was required to give the traditional "Message to the Parents." Everyone in town was in the audience, all three hundred. They all knew my father had just died. I tried to give a tribute to my dad. I was devastated and frozen in grief. Everyone was crying. My graduation turned into another funeral!

So began a long string of negative physical conditions, and I was forced to deal with issues of health and healing on a very dramatic level. I don't know why I created so many illnesses in my body during the following years. Maybe it was because I had always been around sick people as a child and I had been unconsciously programmed to repeat the pattern. I used to ride my bike to visit the sick and elderly in our town. Perhaps I was trying to manifest illnesses to learn about disease. Maybe I had a lot of past-life karma or something and my death urge got activated. Maybe I was full of anger toward God about death and dying issues. Maybe my strong ego needed to be tamed. Maybe my mission in life was to become a healer and master the art of self-healing.

In my adult life, I have created the following illnesses: insomnia, fourteen years of migrating pains, severe hair loss, severe food neurosis, acute arthritis, severe sinusitis, acute hypothermia, melanoma, severe gastritis, rheumatism, paralysis over my heart chakra, a few near-death experiences, and a few other various and sundry ailments. I healed these conditions mostly with my mind and alternative methods, except on two occasions when I was so afraid that I lost my faith in spiritual healing. On those two occasions, I turned to modern medicine, but I eventually realized that my fear had great power over my physical health. My life has been one healing lesson after another, and I hope this book will be of value to others who are on the same journey of self-healing and Physical Immortality. I have learned that all illnesses—even death—are conditions that human beings have created for one reason or another. My healing journey has led me closer to understanding the source of these conditions.

Insomnia

After my father died, I left for my freshman year in college. I was determined to take premed and become a nurse, and I was determined to make straight A's. I had a scholarship to Augustana College, a church college in Sioux Falls, South Dakota. At Augustana, the students had to attend service at the chapel every day. But all I could do was stand outside the chapel and cry. And I could not sleep. I was afraid to shut my eyes—afraid I would wake up dead. I really believed I would die in my sleep. I simply did not sleep. I rarely told anyone about my condition. No one would have believed it anyway, because I still managed to get straight A's. I was always trying to prove myself. It all took its toll, finally, when I began to experience high fevers. I was put in a local hospital, and the college called my mother. The doctors told her they could not find anything wrong with me whatsoever. Once again, I seemed to be manifesting another psychosomatic illness. (Later I would find out that *all* illness is *mental* illness.) The doctors asked us both if we were willing for me to go into therapy. I had one therapy session with a psychiatrist who put me under hypnosis. After the session, he informed both my mother and me that I was not disturbed enough to warrant his high fees. Bless his honest heart! He suggested that I might need group therapy to share with other people my feelings about my father's death. (Had my cats been with me, I surely would have been okay.)

So I went to group therapy. I did okay with it for a while until one of the men there, a minister's son, asked me out for a date. He took me to see the movie *Suddenly Last Summer* starring Elizabeth Taylor. Tennessee Williams is pretty intense, and during the movie, I noticed that my date was gripping the arms of the seat as if he were flipping out. When the movie ended, he informed me that he was going back in to see it again, leaving me standing there alone. So much for my first date in college. The next day he was admitted to a psychiatric ward! I went to see him and his father, the minister, was there. "So much for religion," I thought. Religion had failed again and I was really confused.

That summer I worked as a waitress at the Stanley Hotel in Estes Park, Colorado. Keeping busy and serving others healed me. Apparently, four thousand applications had been submitted by college students, and only thirty were hired by the hotel. I had not even filled out an application. I got the personnel staff's attention by sending them a letter with an explanation of why I thought they should hire me. Even though I was an emotional mess, my higher self was working. (Who wants to sort through four thousand applications?) Once I started to have fun and become more comfortable with sharing my feelings, I quickly got over insomnia.

Amoebic Dysentery and Acute Cystitis

I finally rebelled and left the church school and went off to the University of Florida College of Nursing. I went there for two reasons: First, I could get longer summers off, which allowed me to work to pay college expenses. Second, it was the second biggest party school in the nation, according to *Playboy* magazine. I was fed up with the religious and medical dogma of the Midwest. I needed to relax and have some fun! To be able to attend classes in Bermuda shorts and thongs was mind-blowing. I felt I had experienced a miracle in my life.

In a short time, I met a young man who became my husband, a real genius and adventurer. He was an atheist, which was perfect for me. I did not understand the dynamics of it all then, but I was angry with God about my father's long illness and death. I was in love and we married right after my graduation. We were both inspired by President Kennedy to join the Peace Corps. You could say it was my boot camp training into world service. Our first assignment was Peru. I was very happy, and we both felt we were rebelling against the established norms and making a real difference in the world at the same time. It was a dream come true—to travel and serve others.

We had a tough assignment in Chimbote, Peru. It had almost never rained there in modern history. There were squatter settlements everywhere—and no bathrooms! Our hut had no roof per se, only a makeshift pole-and-straw cover. There was no electricity and no running water. People went to the bathroom in front of everyone, right in the street. It did not bother me that much to see men peeing in the street in front of our hut, but to see them with their pants pulled down, squatting, was another thing. At least the women were covered by their long skirts. Just to cook healthy meals was an ordeal. I had to pressure-cook everything on the Primus stove. It was a real adventure, for sure, and I was determined to see it through.

Before long, we both developed amoebic dysentery despite our preventive efforts. We used to lay in bed and analyze which of us had the worst cramps and who had the most diarrhea. Even though we had been prepared for the possibility of this illness, blood in our stools was a scary thing, even for a nurse. Eventually, my husband lost his hair. He had developed a much rarer and stronger form of the amoeba.

I was not prepared for an acute attack of severe pain in my kidneys and blood in my urine. It was like urinating razor blades. I recognized the symptoms from my nursing books: honeymoon cystitis. It was excruciating. One did not dare consider going to a hospital in that town. The beds had no sheets and filth was everywhere. I had been taking care of babies in that hospital in the worst conditions, and I had seen many babies die of illness and starvation. Plague epidemics were on the rise, and so my husband wired Lima. A Peace Corps helicopter came to evacuate me.

Somehow the word got out that I was really sick. I did not think I was so sick at the time. I just had IVS and thought I was going to be fine. Many of the Peace Corps volunteers heard I was dying and left their posts to visit me. Despite the rumors, I recovered for the time being; but the condition continued and became more chronic later. Many times during my marriage, it got so bad that I ended up hospitalized, needing dilation and other treatments. Sometimes I had to stay on Macrodantin for a year at a time. I became afraid of sex. It ruined my and my husband's sex life. The medical profession could not cure me of this condition. I was a nurse in those days, and I had no idea of alternative healing methods.

My husband and I ended up getting a divorce, and I began to have fewer problems with cystitis and more sexual experiences. What was it about my husband? I know now that I had not experienced any form of enlightenment during my marriage because I was stuck on conventional medical concepts. Also, I knew nothing about the ideas of past lives and karma. The whole experience remained a mystery to me until I realized that I developed cystitis only with certain types of men.

Then one day I met Leonard Orr and I learned about breathwork. I became more conscious of the metaphysical, and I started getting serious about alternative healing. It was not until I had experienced several LRTs that I was able to crack the cystitis case completely.

Once before a training session in Boston, I had a very frightening dream that five men came into my room and left a tarantula on the bed. I woke, terrified and screaming. The next morning at the coffee shop, five men came in and sat down with me at my table. I panicked but tried to remain calm. During the sex therapy section of the training, I nearly fainted. Fortunately, my trainer continued with the session. I pulled out a piece of paper and did some automatic writing: "Five men, rape, Africa." After that, I found myself on the floor in spontaneous breathwork.

Was my ex-husband one of those men? Some alternative healers have found that when we are younger, we often are attracted to past-life mates with whom we have karmic experiences that need to balance out. We must do this before we can move on to more loving and whole relationships. The day after the session in Boston, I happened to have an appointment with a famous aura reader. She told me I had almost totally worked out that karma. Prior to that, I had never understood how past-life experiences could come back to inflict our current bodies. I had healed from cystitis, though. *It was a matter of bringing up the cause and letting it go!*

Fourteen Years of Migrating Pain

In addition to insomnia, I began to experience a lot of physical pain in my body after my father died. This condition developed right after I saw my father in his casket. The pains were intense at times, and they migrated around my body. The whole experience was unusual for me, because prior to my father's dying, I hadn't had any pains. I realized that it was all psychosomatic, and I knew that "doctors" could not help me. I learned to live with those pains for fourteen years until I began breathwork. After three sessions, the mysterious pains left my body and never returned. It was a question of breathing out the "death urge" that had been taken in from my family and activated in me. Now you can understand why I became a breathworker!

Severe Hair Loss

My hair was always naturally curly. In fact, it had gotten so curly while I was in Florida that I bought some hair straightener and almost ruined my hair. But that was nothing compared to what happened to my hair after my divorce. It began falling out to the point that I had a large bald spot and I had to wear a wig to hide it. The more worried I got, the more hair I lost. I was a nurse, so I had access to the best doctors. I went to so many that it became ridiculous, but none of them could help me. I was in constant therapy, but that did not help me either. I was desperate and I was really scared. This all happened prior to my first breathwork experience and my metaphysical awakening. I was still deeply entrenched in the modern medical approach to healing. Nothing worked for me and I became suicidal, which made it even worse.

One day in Phoenix, I visited yet one more dermatologist. I decided he would be the final one. He had white hair and was a sweet father figure. I trusted him. He suggested that I save the amount of hair that fell out each week, put it into a sack, and bring it to him. He wanted to study the amounts to determine if it increased or decreased. It always increased, and the sacks got fuller.

One week he looked at me and said, "My dear, you have a very serious problem."

"You're telling me!" I shrieked. "You are my last hope. I cannot stand to go to another doctor."

He went to his prescription book and wrote down the following: "Go read this book: *Peace of Mind* by Rabbi Leiberman."

I was shocked. "What kind of prescription is this?" I wondered. I read the book and was blown away. It was my first real exposure to metaphysical philosophy. It explained how the mind rules the body. Why hadn't any of the nursing books I had studied covered this? I will always be grateful to the man. My hair stopped falling out, but I still had quite a bald spot. I was starting my third year of this condition.

I remember looking into the mirror and thinking, "What if this never ends?" I had to deal with this fear every single day. But after one straight year of breathwork, I worked out almost all the tension that prevented my hair from becoming healthy. I had some help at that time from my friend, Dr. Irv Katz. He did a couple of hypnotic sessions with me. I really trusted him, for he was a fellow breathworker, LRT graduate, sex therapist, and a great psychologist. He got me right down to all my unconscious issues of loss. Between the breathwork and the sessions with Dr. Katz, I was healed. My hair grew back! It was a miracle for me, and my friends could not believe it. I went on a marvelous trip to Hawaii and was finally free of that condition. The whole experience was a powerful lesson for me.

Isn't it amazing how the issues of loss from my childhood mani-fested into a real, physical condition of loss in my body? My mind, conscious or unconscious, really did rule my body!

Food Neurosis

I was born on the kitchen table, so maybe my food neurosis started then. My birth trauma was all wired up with food. In one of my past-life regression experiences, I found out I had been poisoned by some food. Maybe it all started then. I was always neurotic about food, even as a child. I was terrified of getting fat, and I ate like a bird. To gain even five pounds drove me insane. It was my own pri-vate and inner hell.

My mother was a home economics teacher, and we lived in the heart of the Midwest, where most of the nation's food is grown. Everyone at home was obsessed with food. Well, it seemed that way to me, anyway. In the morning, you get up, think about breakfast, prepare breakfast, eat breakfast, and then clean up after breakfast. Then you think about lunch, prepare lunch, eat lunch, and clean up after lunch. You go through the whole cycle for dinner and even a bedtime snack. My mother was always concerned with food—what to eat with what. The only fights we ever had were in the kitchen and were about food—what to cook or how to prepare it. And then there was the fact that my father took twelve different pills at every single meal. He laid them all out on his plate, which always reminded me of his illness and that he might be dying. I wanted to get out of there and away from the obsession with food.

At one point in my life, I got so neurotic about eating that I actu-ally began to fear eating off my own plate. This got especially intense when my past-life stuff was coming up. I became increas-ingly paranoid and had to eat off one of my friends' plates. Fortunately, most of my friends were very understanding. They would tell me to take a walk around the block or something, which helped me get a grip on myself.

In the late seventies, my neurosis came to a head while visiting my guru Babaji in India. Once, in his presence, I became very nerv-ous and obsessed with the subject of food. I was not overweight at all, but I was constantly worried about it. I lived on the edge of anorexia all the time, but it was ridiculous for me to experience those fears in Babaji's ashram. I decided to confess my obsession to him, for I was, literally, on the verge of severe neurosis. One day I walked right up to him and said, "Babaji, I am totally obsessed and neurotic about the topic of food."

He looked at me and abruptly said, "Oh, just give up food," and then he walked away.

I took this very seriously. Was he implying that I should become a Breatharian and be like Saint Teresa Newman who ate only one communion wafer a day for twenty-five years? I went back to Babaji and asked him if he meant immediately.

"No," he said, "the food here is holy and blessed. You give up food when you go back to America."

I was still a neophyte around Babaji. I took everything that he said literally. I did not understand his ways, his methods, or his *lilas* (divine tricks or play by the master to help you crack your problems). What followed then was really difficult. I began to go nuts, and I tried to imagine never eating again. I was not a vegetarian at the time, and I began to have visions of sizzling steaks going right by the temple and in the presence of Babaji. Then I would see large pizzas, dripping with cheese. These visions were in vivid color and kept getting stronger. I could no longer pray, chant, or meditate. I was losing my mind.

Finally, one evening I knelt before Babaji and once again told the truth: "I've gone crazy now."

Suddenly, he picked up two large cymbals, the kind that one sees in a marching band. He raised them up over my head and crashed them together as hard as he could. My body shook wildly and then it was over. My mind cleared completely. Babaji had given me some type of "sound healing." Later I realized I had never seen those cymbals around him before that moment, nor did I see them any time thereafter. Had he materialized a set of cymbals for my healing? Was it all a dream?

And yet, still taking Babaji literally, when I left India, I gave up food as he had told me to do. He had also told me to walk every morning at 4 A.M. I was in Hawaii and I gave up food for thirty days. Every morning I got up and walked. I was not hungry, but I felt very angry. I had to take long walks to clear the anger. After thirty days of this routine, I realized it was all just a *lila*, and the whole point of it all was for me to process some of my anger about death. I started to feel better and eat normally.

There were a few setbacks, though. I was fine until some of my friends and I piled into a car and drove to Mexico for a lobster feed. We were on a beach with mariachis playing, and unlimited amounts of lobster just kept coming and coming. I wondered how my friends could eat so much and still be so happy. I reached my limit right away, and then all my fear came up again. On the way home from that trip, I curled up in the fetal position and prayed to Babaji and Jesus for liberation. I pleaded once again for help. Then I heard the words *"the only diet there is,"* and I realized I was being told to write another book.

Other than this book, *The Only Diet There Is* was the hardest book I ever wrote. One-third of the way through, I got severe writer's block and could not write anything for a year. I was really struggling. But thanks to my friend R. R. who was a brilliant restaurateur, I broke through. He could eat any amount of food without gaining weight or getting full. I picked his brain and his secrets worked. I dedicated that book to him. I was finally able to break through my writer's block and my food neurosis condition—and I was able to finish the book. "The Ego and Food" chapter really put it all together. Afterward it did not matter what I ate, and I stopped thinking about the whole issue. I had always wanted to be able to eat anything and not gain weight. By the time I really achieved that, I was bored with food altogether. I was finally liberated. It felt like heaven to be free of that ridiculous pattern.

Acute Arthritis

All of my healing issues were beginning to dissolve as I came deeper into metaphysical understanding. I was beginning to feel really good. It was a thrill to be at the beginning of breathwork and studying with Leonard Orr. I was over my divorce, had a new boyfriend, and we were in San Francisco during the heyday of the alternative consciousness movement. We lived in a spiritual community, and Leonard Orr was teaching us the concepts of Physical Immortality. I had already been working out my unconscious death urges the hard way, so I adapted quickly to Leonard's ideas. I wanted to live and I wanted to be healthy. I was ecstatic to learn that I may be able to prolong my life. I gave up nursing and modern medicine that year. One day I just walked out. Why should I stay in a profession that did not produce the quick and *Permanent Healings* that I was seeing in breathwork? (See "Breathworking and Healing" on page 106.)

I was so enthusiastic about breathwork that I told Leonard I thought I should write a book for breathworkers and include all the information on Physical Immortality. Most of that information was underground, and I was beginning to find out. I felt that my second book should be called Breathworking in the New Age. I wanted to write it with Leonard, and I told him that we needed a chapter on Physical Immortality. That night we tossed the I Ching to see if the world was ready for such a book. The I Ching came out with the following: "Yes, but you are on very thin ice." We decided to write it.

I locked myself in seclusion and began the chapter on Physical Immortality. I had no idea how much would come up from my subconscious mind. I was in a bit over my head. It was still a radical thing to discuss these subjects. A few days into it, my fingers locked up with gripping pain. I ran into Leonard's room crying hysterically.

"Leonard," I shouted, "I have arthritis!" I knew I could have a brilliant writing career, and I was barely getting started. Now it might all be over!

He looked at me calmly and said, "Oh, this is great!"

"What do you mean?" I screamed at him. "How can this be great?"

Then he said it was great because I was going through my old age early and that he did not have to worry about me anymore. He was not concerned at all. I began to relax. Only an Immortal could have gotten me through that moment. I began breathwork feverishly for three weeks to process out the arthritis. It worked! Breathwork had healed me again.

The important thing I learned is that we need to be in the presence of enlightened friends who do not go into agreement with our negative conditions. If Leonard had gotten as upset as I had, I would have been sunk and most likely would have arthritis to this day. This is exactly how Jesus healed people. He never affirmed their egos; he only saw them healed. I went through several early aging releases after that.

Leonard Orr once said, "It is better to go through that stuff when you are young and strong enough to really process it."

Severe Sinusitis

I was in Bali with close associates and friends. It was my birthday, and we were all having a great time. That afternoon I developed a sudden sinus block without any warning. I had not been sick for a long time, and I thought it would just pass. It did not pass, and later I realized that it started at the exact time of my birth, 2:30 in the afternoon, August 24. It took me awhile to put the connection together. I continued to travel, and the condition kept getting worse, especially because I was flying in airplanes a lot. I went from healer to healer and worked on myself constantly. By then, I had learned how to clear my mind much better, but it did not work on my sinus infection. Nothing I did helped, nor were the healers I visited able to clear the problems. When it finally sunk in that the condition really started at the exact time of my birth, I called Dr. Bob Doughten, the only obstetrician in the States who was also a breathworker. He had actually been breathworking teenagers whom he had delivered years before! That really impressed me, and I was anxious to see him.

I flew to Portland, where he lived, and I suggested that he breathwork me on the kitchen floor since I was born in the kitchen. He was more than willing. It is great to have a good breathworker, but it is the ultimate to have an obstetrician breathwork you. Wow! There is nothing like that! I told him I thought I needed to review my whole birth one more time. I asked him to imagine pulling me out. He put his hands on my head while I breathed. Then he suddenly said, "Oh, I see they pulled you out wrong."

I felt pain around my nose and shouted, "I am damaged!" I reexperienced my sinus area being nearly crushed by the doctor who had delivered me.

I had stopped the birth process myself, waiting for my father to come back into the kitchen. He had gone out to the porch to light a cigarette! That is when the doctor tried to pull me out, but I wanted to wait a little longer. (Cigarettes had affected my whole life!) I remembered the whole scenario then and there.

Dr. Doughten sat me up, looked into my eyes, and said, "You know that you have the power to heal this yourself, but you are not doing it. You are setting your life up in such a way that you have to go back to modern medicine so that you are forced to forgive doctors."

I knew he was right. Large tears flew out of my eyes toward his eyes, and I promised him I would go.

In Denver, I opened the phone book to professional specialists in ENT. I ran my finger down the page, and it stopped at Dr. Roy Jones. The only appointment I could get was at 2:30 in the afternoon, the exact time of my birth! I walked into his office and almost fell over. He looked exactly like Dr. Moore, my obstetrician! I could not believe it. I thought that it all had to be a Babaji *lila,* and I told my assistant Wendy to help me surrender to this doctor totally. I was not going to fight anything that he said.

When he came back with the X rays, he said, "These are opaque four. I cannot possibly let you leave here without surgery! You must avoid flying, and you are very lucky that you don't have optic nerve damage. I just cannot believe you have been walking around with this condition."

So there it was. Did I dare confess to him my arrogance, that I thought I would never need a doctor again and that I had no insurance? He was very kind and understanding when I told him the truth. He arranged it so I could go in as an outpatient and go home right after the surgery.

The last thing I ever wanted to do was to go back to modern medicine, but I remembered what Dr. Bob Doughten had said and I humbled myself. The whole ordeal turned into a very spiritual experience. The nurses had somehow read my books. They were like angels. The surgeon introduced me to the anesthesiologist, saying that they had an excellent relationship and had gone to school together. While I was in the waiting room, the surgeon came out and called my name. He said that my surgery went very well!

I thought I was losing it for a moment and said, "Wait a minute, I have not even gone in yet!"

He seemed confused and ruffled. Was he channeling my name or the outcome of the as-yet-unperformed surgery? I took it as a message from Babaji that everything was going to be okay. I went into the operating room relaxed. Apparently, while under anesthesia, I gave everyone in the room a very clear lecture on how dolphins were programmed by Atlanteans. They were all amazed, and I hear they still talk about it.

Later I visited a healer in Madrid who was very strong but said little. I told him nothing about my ordeal. He passed his hand over my sinus area and said only, "Karmic break."

Then I saw that I had allowed myself to be experimented on with some type of lasers in ancient Atlantis . . . something to do with the uplifting of humanity. (I can imagine myself doing that!)

The whole experience of severe sinusitis taught me that many, if not all, of our physical conditions are absolutely linked to our past. Whether it be past lives, birth traumas, or childhood conditioning, our illnesses and physical problems are almost always rooted in some form of negative, unconscious memory that we can discover and release through breathwork and other methods of alternative healing.

Acute Hypothermia

I took time off from my own healing journey and went home to see my sister shortly before she died of melanoma. Her aura was quite gray and she was very angry. I spent hours with her while she vented her feelings. I tried to help her as much as I could. I gave her lists of people who had healed themselves of cancer. I gave her lists of healers who had actually been successful healing people with cancer. I hoped that she would ask for help—but to no avail. She had not even read my books! I was a heretic in her eyes. When she flat-out refused to read the lists, I was devastated.

When I left her that last time, I began to experience intense cold and freezing chills throughout my body. Apparently, I was channeling as much of my family's death urge as I could stand, which triggered more of my own. I shook and shook and could not get warm, no matter what I did. The cold got so intense that when I walked into a room, the heat from the venting systems turned cold and the hot water in the taps did the same. It happened several times, even in my friend Fred's room. He was a personal witness to this bizarre phenomenon.

I could not shake the chills. Even when I wore a warm coat at the airports, people walked up to me and told me I looked cold! Finally, I decided that a trip to the hot springs in California was in order. By a small miracle, I attracted a polarity therapist who was able to teach me how to treat my condition. He told me to stay in the hot thermal water as long as I could stand it and then go directly into cold water. I could not imagine plunging into cold water, but he said it would "set the heat" in my bones. I followed his instructions and it worked. I was able to connect with Mother Nature and heal through another bout with that old death urge.

Melanoma

About six months after my sister died, I was in New Delhi with my then boyfriend. He was a yogi who had spent about ten years in India. Before that, he had been a "doctor." By the grace of Babaji, he was there with me. He happened to notice a mole on my left leg, and he told me it was serious and needed to be removed. I had not even noticed anything wrong; it looked like an ordinary mole to me. I was working hard to tune out illness and my past connections with ordinary medicine—not dwell on them. I could tell he was channeling, and I figured I better listen to him. When we returned to the States, I went to get it checked. Sure enough, it was melanoma. I was shocked; I was not the cancer type at all. Was I going into sympathy with my sister? Was it my last-ditch approach to win her love by being like her and manifesting the same death symptoms?

It turned out that the melanoma was not very deep, and they were able to get it all.

Then, exactly one year after my sister's death, I was in Atlanta. I went into a major death trauma or something and threw myself on the bed while screaming, "I want to live! I want to live!"

I called my friend Rhonda to help me. For four days, I went through intense paranoia about dying, and I did not want to be alone. There was nothing wrong with me physically whatsoever. Rhonda's son was there, and he had happened to cut himself and needed to see a doctor. I went with them and mentioned my fear condition to the doctor.

When I told him it had been exactly one year since my sister died, he asked me, "Don't you know that it is very common for family members to have strong delayed reactions one year after a loved one's death?" Somehow his words cleared me.

Later I was in Bali again, and I was having a wonderful time. But one night I woke up having a horrible nightmare. I saw my sister and she was deranged. I woke up screaming and saw that another spot of skin cancer on my leg had popped up overnight! I was confused and could not understand what was going on. I went to my altar and started praying. I was not about to go to a doctor in Indonesia. My next stop on the trip was India, where I went to see a doctor who was a Babaji devotee. He looked up at the pictures of our guru and said, "Let's see what the old master has in store for you."

He called the chief surgeon of Delhi who had treated the president of India. That doctor was one of the best available and had studied in London. Okay, I could handle that. The clinic was marginal, but I trusted him. He told me I needed to have it removed quickly just in case it was malignant. I was not going to mess around with melanoma. That form of cancer can move very fast. I decided to go ahead with the surgery and process my mind later.

Fortunately, I was on my way to Rajastan to see my guru Shastriji. I cried at his feet and begged him to explain what was going on with me. What he said to me then gave me the shock of my life.

He said, "I regret to tell you, but your sister has not crossed over properly. She has been entering your body to get attention because she knows that you are the only one advanced enough to help her."

"What?" I asked. "How can this be?" These weird things could not possibly happen to *my* family. "Is he talking about possession?" I wondered.

He told me I had to follow his instructions exactly, and that if it didn't work, I would have to go to Banares—the place where souls cross over. Banares . . . I could not believe it! Shastriji also told me I had to immediately chant five thousand mantras for her and perform a fine ceremony. Then I would have to perform a ceremony in the Ganges for the dead and wait to see if my sister would appear to me again. I did exactly what my guru instructed, but let me tell you, it was one of the hardest tasks in my life.

I had never tried five thousand mantras before. I did one thousand a day for five days. I focused almost all my attention toward my sister. While in Delhi, I became terrified at the thought of not being able to complete what Shastriji had instructed me to do to help my sister. What if her soul were lost in the cosmos for thousands of years? I got really scared and cried for hours. At one point, I was so upset that I had to go next door to the hotel room of my friends, Carmen and Adolfo. I got in bed with the whole family, and they held me while I worked on my breathing. Adolfo was my perfect breathworker. He shared with me how his brother had died in his arms from an overdose of drugs.

My "group," which consisted of students coming from all over the world to train with me in India, was about to arrive at the hotel at any time. I had to recover! I put all my soul into that breathwork, finished my mantras, and all the fear cleared just five minutes before I had to meet my students. Later I performed the ceremonies just as Shastriji had instructed. My sister appeared to me, and she seemed all right. I obviously had something to work out and clear with her to stop manifesting cancer in my body. I went to a few past-life therapists and reviewed all my karma with my sister. I received amazing information. If I had not worked through all of that and released it, I surely would have struggled with more bouts of cancer over and over. As of today, I have been completely healed of melanoma!

After that ordeal, I found peace with my issues about modern medicine. Many times people have a lot of fear about self-healing and must therefore rely on doctors for help. Self-healing can be a deep and complicated issue, and we all need help to make the gradual transition to alternative healing methods. But I have found that prayer helps and that through prayer, we can always attract the perfect healers in our life when we need them.

Rheumatism

After my first experience of writing a chapter on Physical Immortality (when I got arthritis), I was terrified of the prospect of writing a whole book on the subject. It took me nine years to get up the courage. I did not have a computer in those days. When I finally decided it was time to tackle this project, I bought a new electric typewriter. To my dismay, the typewriter kept blowing up, and I had to keep taking it back.

"Ma'am," the man at the store said, "you're too powerful. You have to upgrade."

I had to keep upgrading until I ended up with the absolutely most expensive model they had (of course). But then the lights in my flat started blowing out, and a lot of strange things began to happen. I was busy writing, and I didn't let it bother me that much. It felt as though other forces were at work around me and coming through me. There was a force of resistance as well but, somehow, I got through it.

When I called my mother to tell her that I had written the most important manuscript of my life, I felt so happy and *alive*. It was during that same phone call that I first found out about my sister's cancer. All of the joy I had been feeling immediately drained out of me. Shortly afterward, the book was released. I remember when I saw the first hardback edition: I was signing books in Los Angeles, and the line for autographs was longer than I had ever experienced. As the line finally got toward the end, I felt a very strange reaction in my body. Suddenly, I felt extremely odd and heavy as lead.

The next morning I was preparing to give a speech on the subject of Physical Immortality at a local Los Angeles church. While I was dressing, I suddenly experienced a sensation of shattering glass in my left hip, and I fell to the floor. The pain was terrible. I crawled to the phone and called a friend who was an excellent psychic. I pleaded with him to tell me what was happening. He said that the topic of my presentation was opposed to that which the church usually teaches and that I was meeting some real resistance. I told him I was going despite whatever was blocking me. I cried in the taxi all the way to the church. There was no doubt that I was having a spontaneous breathwork session.

When I arrived at the church, I immediately told the staff I needed to lie down. "How much time do I have?" I asked.

"Twenty minutes. And the only place to lie down is in the kitchen," someone said. This was perfect, of course, for I was born in the kitchen!

Some of the breathworkers in the audience saw me coming in, realized I was in trouble, and got up to help me. I was crying and breathing like mad, trying to get ready for my talk, but the time ran out. Someone opened the swinging door and shouted, "You're on!"

My eye makeup was running down my face, my suit was wrinkled, and I could hardly walk. My body felt like old age was setting in and fast. It was clear to me that I had developed the symptoms of rheumatism. I had to be helped all the way to the stage. I was a mess and hardly in any kind of shape to give a lecture on *How to Be Chic, Fabulous, and Live Forever.* I told the audience that I had to go through this in front of them. People started crying in the audience, and some of them went into spontaneous breathwork sessions right there. Imagine their meeting me for the first time while I was in that condition!

Suddenly, my energy shifted and I gave a brilliant lecture on the *"Immortals of the Bible."* I don't remember any of it except the fact that I was given a standing ovation. After that, I ended up right back on the kitchen floor in pain. I stayed on a couch most of the afternoon, unable to move.

I remembered that two days before, someone had put the phone number of an acupuncturist whom they liked in my coat pocket. That was one of the little miracles that has kept me going as a public figure. I went for a treatment, and it helped me a lot. At least I was able to get on my feet and walk. But for the next few days, when I visited my breathwork clients in Hollywood, I had to hobble up to those mansions like a little old lady. It was really embarrassing. On top of it all, I had to go to Australia in that condition. For three whole weeks, I had severe symptoms of rheumatism. I had chiropractic treatments and all kinds of other treatments. When I got back to the States, I called my mother to ask her how she was.

"Oh," she said, "I had a real bad spell with my hip these past weeks but now it's gone."

Later that day my hip suddenly healed, and I have not had the problem since. What was it with my family and me? Was my health that psychically connected to theirs? Was this their stuff or mine?

After that experience, I became really confused about all my strange physical conditions and my sensitivity to other people's illnesses and death. I knew Babaji could process other people's stuff and worlds of karma through his body all the time, but he knew how to do it. I was obviously not very good at it. I began to wonder where the boundaries of my being were.

Gastritis

I was working in Berlin shortly after the Wall came down. I was very sensitive to all the personal and social trauma that surrounded it all. It so happened that my two nieces were in Germany, and my mother came to visit all of us. There we were, meeting together for the first time since my sister died. I had just found out that my niece had been pregnant when her mother (my sister) passed on. The baby was born with mild problems. We were all emotional wrecks, and it was all just too much for me. I could not digest it and I could not digest Berlin. Out of nowhere, I developed a terrible pain in my upper intestines. I could not eat and I wondered if I had manifested an ulcer.

Like so many times before, I was privileged to have a wonderful assistant who was actually an obstetrician. She was amazing—also a trained breathworker and a rock star! She was fun to be around and cheered me up.

For the first time in quite a while, I really had a chance to talk with my mother. I asked her if I had suffered with colic or something as an infant.

To my shock, she said, "Yes . . . for six weeks."

I asked why I had colic and she said, "Oh, some babies have colic and some don't."

That answer did not satisfy me at all. I told her it had probably been caused by cow's milk and that I thought I was angry that she had not breast-fed me. She was understanding and agreed that maybe I was right.

Later I asked my assistant breathworker to give me a deep session on the issue of breast-feeding. I went back to the time of my infancy and found that I had feelings and preverbal thoughts that translated to something like this: "I can never forgive this. They might as well put me out in the street!" I was really angry that I had not been breast-fed. No wonder I had suffered with colic as an infant, and no wonder I had developed gastritis as an adult.

I started to pray very hard to Babaji. I cried at my altar and pleaded with him to help me. I wondered how I was going to do a whole European tour when I could not even eat. Then a miracle happened. I was doing a seminar with mostly German people. An Italian man walked in late. I could not understand what he was doing there, and I wondered if he could understand German or the translation into English.

At the break, we ended up in the same elevator, and he introduced himself as Michelangelo.

I suddenly blurted out, "Oh, you are the one for Italy. Please come to my room after we finish." I was startled at myself for being so direct. The words just came out of my mouth, but I had learned before to trust these things. He seemed to have no problem with it at all.

He came to my room later. He was a divine being and an angel. To my amazement, he told me he was a devotee of Babaji and Muniraj. I was astonished. He told me he had been *called* to come, that he had actually been in a car wreck on the way, but felt he still had to make it to the seminar. It turned out to be another Babaji miracle for me. I felt compelled to tell him about my condition, and he said he could help. He pulled some very fine, high-vibration food out of his bag. It looked like vegetable pâté and baby food. He fed me as if I were an infant, and I was able to eat a little. My prayers had been answered.

He told me he could heal me in two weeks if I could travel to Milan. It was a nice idea but I had a whole tour to complete, so I could not arrange to get away. The rest of the trip, I managed to eat a teaspoon of bee pollen each day and a few fresh dates while in Spain. I was unable to eat anything else, literally.

During this period, people began telling me I needed to take time off, which was the last thing I wanted to hear. I was a workaholic who could not stop. But then a funny thing happened: perfect strangers started walking up to me on the street and telling me I needed to take time off. This happened so many times that I realized Babaji must be speaking to me through other people and that I better wake up.

I canceled part of my tour and rented a cottage on Cape Cod. Then I sent Michelangelo a plane ticket, for he had agreed to come and stay with me for a few weeks. The day before he came, I decided to ask him to shave my head. I was in trouble with my body, and I wanted to facilitate the maximum healing possible in the manner I had learned from my gurus in India. I called my mother to tell her how happy I was with my decision. I had done this before, so I thought she could handle it this time, but she was not happy at all. It was the one thing about my spiritual journey that was just too much for her. Besides, she had made plans for me to visit relatives, and she didn't think it would be good for them to see me that way. I told her I would just not go and that my healing would have to take top priority. It was hard, but it was all I could do. I knew she would get over it in time, but would I ever get over my stomach condition if I did not take some time for myself? I wanted to be in optimum cooperation with whatever Michelangelo wanted to do. I had to surrender.

I prepared an altar in my cottage. Then I fixed a basket with all the necessities for the head shaving *(mundun)*. I covered the basket with a sacred cloth and put it under the altar. I even called an astrologer to ask when the perfect time would be. She was astonished that the time I had chosen was absolutely perfect—the Fourth of July—and she suggested one minute before midnight.

That night one of my students picked up Michelangelo at the airport and drove him to my cottage. It was good to see him. I immediately told him about my desire, and he was agreeable to the idea. He had absolutely no problem accepting the sacred responsibility. After all, he had his head shaved several times, and he understood the deep meaning and power this type of healing gives.

We started the *mundun* one minute before midnight. It took quite awhile and I was awake all night. I had shaved my head twice before, and I thought a third time would be a snap. But I was shocked at how spiritually strong it was. I lay on the couch for days feeling my energy chakras swirling around and around. It was a very strange sensation, and I felt as though I were turning inside out.

Michelangelo began giving me hour-and-a-half sessions of reflexology twice a day. He is a master and his touch was very intense. He also prepared and fed me his high-vibration foods each day. It was hard for me to digest even little amounts, but I managed to get down small portions. After about ten days, I began to have a real healing crisis and started to go kind of berserk. He helped me by taking me for long walks and making me walk faster and faster, which got my breathing into a constant breathwork mode. The final week he took some time to go to one of my LRTs in Connecticut. It was my gift to him. When he came back, he was excited but had gone through an energy shift himself. He ended up on the floor, breathing through his own healing crisis before he went back to Italy!

By the end of his visit, I was much better. I left Cape Cod and went to Bali for a rest. It was wonderful to be on that island and with a shaved head! I was so glad I had taken some time for self-healing, and I was so grateful to Michelangelo.

After Bali, I went to India. I wanted to give my thanks and prayers to Babaji. While I was in the Himalayas, I met a beautiful Dutch man. We really hit it off and both felt we had been together in a past life as young lovers in Poland. Well, it just so happened that I was scheduled to do the first LRT ever given in Poland right after my mission in India. Naturally, my new friend decided to travel with me.

The whole experience of gastritis taught me that an adult healing crisis often directly relates to a childhood or infancy crisis. In my case, I was able to bring up my feelings of lack and anger at not being breast-fed and deal with them. I was able to let them go and receive some special healing before they ate a hole in my body. The symptom is not the illness, nor is it the problem. The source of healing is much deeper and related to the condition of our mental and emotional selves. I can only be eternally grateful that I was able to expand my awareness beyond modern medicine and traditional religion.

The Basics of Metaphysical Healing

- ❖ The mind rules the body.

- ❖ The body is the effect of the mind.

- ❖ Negative thoughts produce negative results in the body.

- ❖ What you think expands in the material/physical world.

- ❖ Anything can be cured. We create illness with our minds, and we can *uncreate* it with our minds.

- ❖ We will give up pain or the symptom when we see no more value in it. *(A Course in Miracles)*

- ❖ The real physician is the mind of the patient. The outcome of healing is what the mind of the patient decides. *(A Course in Miracles)*

- ❖ Disease is often anger taken out on the body.

- ❖ It is an immutable spiritual law that when there is a health problem, there is a forgiveness problem. (Ponder, Catherine. *The Dynamic Laws of Healing.*)

  You have healing power within you. Permanent Healing comes from freeing the mind and health is basically an inside job. The mind is in every cell of your body. Every cell is enveloped in thought. Your body is composed of radiant substance. The body is soft, pliable, and even plastic to your thoughts. (Catherine Ponder)

- ❖ All healing is, essentially, the release from fear. Fear causes pain and disease.

- ❖ Resentment, anger, hate, condemnation, and the desire to get even tear down your body.

- ❖ You are not a victim. There are no victims. Life presents us with whatever our thoughts are—conscious or unconscious.

PART II

Causes of Sickness

*"There is nothing that is incurable except that
which you acknowledge as incurable.*

*"To change your body, all that you have to
do is change your mind and your body
will change automatically."*

LEONARD ORR, FOUNDER OF BREATHWORK

Negative Thoughts
and Personal Lies

Personal lies can make you sick and keep you from healing yourself.

In my other books, I often discuss how our most negative thoughts can affect our lives. These include negative, preverbal thoughts from birth and infancy. In this chapter, I try to show you how these negative thoughts can sabotage our ability to heal ourselves. *Personal laws* or *lies* are our most negative thoughts about ourselves, usually formed at birth, in the womb, or brought in as a core belief from a past life. Originally, we called these thoughts personal laws because we believe them to be true and they can control our whole lives. But because they are not the *real* truth about ourselves, we now emphasize that these thoughts are *personal lies*.

Here are some of the most common personal lies we have seen in breathworking:

I am not good enough.	*I am a failure.*
I am bad.	*Something's wrong with me.*
I am wrong.	*I am a disappointment.*
I am not perfect.	*I shouldn't be here.*
I am weak.	*I am unwanted.*
I am guilty.	*I am evil.*
I can't.	*I am stuck.*
I can't make it.	*I am nothing.*

In everyone we have breathworked, we have been able to find one of the above thoughts predominant. The person's tendency is to act out the negative thought, suppress it, and overcompensate, and/or project it onto someone else. For example, persons with the thought "I am bad" may act bad and do things that are bad, bringing on themselves bad judgment from others and actually reinforcing the thought of badness. Or they may work very hard to keep the thought of being bad completely hidden from other people and overcompensate by acting especially good all the time. They may become obsessed with being good, not seeing that their behavior is only a cover-up. Or, finally, they may project their bad thoughts onto others and start seeing everyone else as bad instead of facing such defects in themselves.

Unfortunately, these thoughts are like addictions. A person believes a thought so strongly that after years and years of accepting it, the thought just seems to be normal. It also feels as though one's life almost totally depends on keeping that thought alive. The person starts believing that is who he or she really is. Having survived both birth and infancy with that thought, the person suffers an unconscious fear that he or she will die if he or she gives up the thought. Of course, this does not make any sense. It is just a trick of the ego.

Some people mistakenly think that as soon as they discover their personal lie, they can drop it overnight. However, people usually fear an overnight shift in habit patterns. They fear too much light or too much of an energy change all at once. Most people tend to chip away at negative thoughts and let them go slowly over time.

These negative thoughts are in the deep subconscious, so most people might not even be aware they have a block unless they experience breathwork or some similar purification technique. The following are examples of how each of these negative thoughts can interfere with healing.

I am not good enough: These people might accept the idea that they are not good enough to be healed. So no matter how many healing opportunities have been given them, none will help, because deep down these people believe they are not good enough to deserve the result of healing. So they will create the *sabotage pattern.*

I am wrong: People who think they are wrong also think they deserve punishment, and the illness may be the very punishment they think they deserve. These people may also attract the *wrong* diagnosis, the *wrong* medicine, the *wrong* doctor or healer, and they never get anywhere. They may even get stuck on working in the wrong part of their mind on the wrong issues.

I am not perfect: These people often make up little things wrong with their bodies so they can feel imperfect. They might be obsessed with the imperfections they create. As soon as they heal one imperfection, they make up another so they can make sure they are never perfect. Often, they are never satisfied with the doctor or healer they choose, projecting that the doctor or healer is imperfect! Even if they should find the perfect doctor or healer, they might set up their treatment so something goes wrong and they can remain imperfect.

I am weak: These people may make up an illness that results in a feeling of weakness. Then they can physically experience the fact that they are weak, thus manifesting the proof that they are weak. They might create an illness such as anemia, for example, or Epstein-Barr virus, chronic fatigue syndrome, or something else that saps their energy. Often, these people are premature at birth and get stuck in the thought "I am too weak to heal myself."

I am guilty: Because guilt demands punishment, this person makes sure he or she is punished somehow. They might become sexually promiscuous so they can continue the guilt cycle and come up with a sexually transmitted disease. They may create something such as herpes out of healthy, normal sex. They may punish themselves in a number of ways—from losing money, friends, or a good job to anything else that feeds the guilt and causes them to suffer. Of course, the most natural way to take out guilt is on the body, and these people may create not getting healed because they feel too guilty to deserve healing.

I can't or *I can't make it:* Sometimes these people create mysterious illnesses or diseases that cannot be diagnosed. They think they absolutely can't be healed. Thoughts of helplessness and despair get stretched out to "I can't let go . . . I can't get rid of this . . . I can't control my body." These people can really get stuck in the thought "I can't let go of the thought, I can't." (Not to worry, trained breathworkers know how to handle these conditions.)

I am a failure: Imagine a person trying to heal himself or herself with the unconscious thought "I am a failure." It won't work! They have set themselves up to fail at self-healing before they even try. Failing repeatedly with the same healing techniques is a typical pattern that this person would manifest to prove the thought "I am a failure." Of course, this pattern brings up the death urge, and their condition will truly get worse fast.

Something is wrong with me: This personal lie is a pretty obvious and sure bet that something wrong will be created in the body. For example, I have known women with fertility problems that had the "Something is wrong with me" syndrome. They ran from doctor to doctor trying to get "proof" of infertility. It drove them nuts if the doctors found nothing wrong. What they did not see was that the infertility problem was a result of their thought, and actually, nothing was wrong at all. I have known women with fertility problems who gave themselves up as hopeless; yet, after they had breathwork and had breathed out that thought, they became pregnant!

I shouldn't be here: This personal lie can really be deadly, because these persons have quite a death urge and may go around creating near-fatal accidents and illnesses. These people more often than not live on the edge of personal disaster. They may go around bragging to others about how many "near misses" with death they have had. Some of the AIDS patients I have breathworked harbored this thought. (This thought can be changed. However, these persons must start thinking they deserve to be alive. It is a drastic shift in energy!) Some of these people have a lot of out-of-body experiences and might even be great clairvoyants. However, when these people get really sick, it can be hard for the doctors trying to keep them on this plane.

I am unwanted: People with this thought pattern are often attracted to people of the opposite sex who are not attracted to them so they can feel unwanted. The sadness of constant rejection can make them feel devastated and sick, of course. The problem is compounded because often they cannot ask for the support they need to be healed; they believe other people do not want to help them since they are unwanted.

I am evil: This is a core belief, usually brought in from a past life or several past lives. People of this type are very hard on themselves and believe they deserve severe punishment. They might unconsciously destroy everything good in their lives—businesses, relationships, and even their bodies. They cannot ever imagine that they might deserve happiness and success. These people usually need a lot of spiritual help. Some women who were former prostitutes have this thought. Even though they may not be prostitutes in this life, they tend to manifest the attributes of one to make others believe they are as evil as they believe themselves to be. It is common for these people to create incurable diseases to keep others away, feeling that they deserve no healing whatsoever.

I am stuck: These people may have actually been stuck in the birth canal. Later they get stuck in all kinds of situations or stuck with an ongoing weight problem. Their minds may go in vicious circles trying to figure out how to change, but they often get nowhere because they get stuck.

I am nothing: These people have very low self-esteem; they may think they deserve nothing. Often they manifest anorexia or other diseases that waste away the body. The sad part is that they almost never reach out for help, for they truly believe that nothing or no one exists out there to help them. They may even turn atheistic and deny the love and support of God and the universe. This is a dangerous negative thought pattern; some of these people really believe they are nothing and that nothing can help them.

Although all of these negative thought patterns seem rather extreme, the truth is that these patterns are more common than most people realize, and breathworkers see them day in and day out. For over two decades, I have watched people wrestle with these deep-rooted thoughts and their effects. To breathworkers, changing these thought patterns is not so grim as it may seem. Breathworkers themselves have gone through their own breathwork, discovered their own personal lies, and have survived. On the other side of these thoughts is a whole new life!

Often we hear of the death of someone who had been a happy, healthy, and positive person. She or he may not even have been very old. People may say, "I just cannot understand why one so healthy died, loving life so much." Even people who appear happy and healthy may have deep-rooted negative thought patterns carried from birth or past lives that silently and secretly run their present lives. Now you might have an insight into a person's early death, or it could be past-life karma, of course. Breathworking might prevent early death!

You could be one of the best healers in the world (and if you are, I salute you and hope to meet you someday), but all your work with a client can go down the drain if the person goes back to his or her addictions and personal lies. For your work to have more lasting or permanent effects, please consider suggesting breathwork to your clients. They will appreciate you all the more, and your healing service will be more valuable in the end. Please also consider breathwork for yourself. Your own healing abilities will greatly improve after you discover your own birth and past-life thought patterns. If you get good results now, imagine what you might get after eliminating your own personal lies.

A well-trained breathworker will go after the personal lies in the first session with a client. For a list of breathworkers in your area call the number in the back of the book.

Family Loyalty

You may think you do not want to copy your parents, especially not their *ailments.* Of course, none of us wants to do that! But we feel a deep loyalty to our parents even if we do not feel close to them. In breathwork, we have seen family loyalty take an unconscious form of copying not only parental behavior problems but also of copying parental illness and death patterns. It is an unconscious process and an unhealthy form of "loving" that does not make any sense at all. People that are natural conformists manifest these patterns frequently. Rebels, on the other hand, are less likely to manifest them. However, everyone is susceptible to family loyalty.

When it come to disease, many people say they inherited theirs. They may believe their disease is genetic and there is nothing they can do about it. But what if we could acknowledge the fact that we *choose* to go into agreement with our parents and the genes of our parents? What if we could change our genes and that parental agreement *with our minds*? You may think this is preposterous, but I know of cases where it has been done!

I once went out with a lawyer from Texas whose whole family had Huntington's chorea. By all odds, he was supposed to have it too. It is a horrible disease of dementia. He told me about the day that he *chose* not to go into agreement with that disease. It was such a powerful experience for him that he could perfectly remember the day and time of his decision. He could remember everything that was in the room where he was at the time—the color and design of the carpet, curtains, and everything. To this day, his family doctors are mystified by his case and can't understand how he beat the odds. He was twelve years old when he made that decision.

Shouldn't this story say something about what we tell our children? If we pass on our negative thoughts to them, they surely will have to struggle to overcome all the potential illness, failure, and unhappiness these thoughts tend to manifest. How do we know when it is too late to change our genes? Is it ever too late? Miracle healings happen all the time and all over the world. I strongly recommend that you read *Quantum Healing* by Dr. Deepak Chopra if you still have doubts about the power of the mind to change the body.

Many people have already unconsciously programmed their own death to match that of a parent, grandparent, or loved one. This perpetuates the notion that you cannot do anything about inherited diseases. The statistics of such diseases then climb higher and higher, and that in turn perpetuates the programming even more. Have you even considered how early we start our conscious and unconscious programming? In my seminars on Physical Immortality, I ask people to write down at what age they think they will die and of what condition. Their answers usually come out quite easily because their decisions were made when they were children! When I ask them why they hold that belief about their death, they often reply that it is because of their first funeral experience or the death of a grandparent or loved one. The conditioning thought was "I guess I will be like him or her." A person can identify with a parent or a grandparent so strongly that they take on that body type—thought process and all.

A person's genetics can change! And I have learned that a person's palm can reveal their genetics. One of my gurus is also a palmist. He reads my palm once every seven years or so because the genetic information changes, according to him. Once I met a man in Russia who had no lines at all on his palm. There was just a little X in the middle. I freaked out! I asked him what it meant.

"Total mutation," he said.

He also told me he had waited all his life to find another person who understood Physical Immortality like I did. (He fell in love with me, but he did not know one word of English and I didn't know Russian!)

Once in a healing seminar that I presented, I had a vision of a new healing process right on the spot: I had two people sit across from each other and record on paper all the symptoms and diseases their mothers had, which of those they had copied, and why they had copied them. Then I had them do the same for their fathers and then for their grandparents. It was a lengthy process that grew so intense that I decided never to do it again unless an immediate breathwork session took place afterward. I found myself personally doing the new process for weeks after that seminar. I processed out all the disease programming that my grandmother had had in her body. Had I not been able to do breathwork each step of the way, I am sure I would have ended up with early, permanent aging. Many times in my life, I had manifested premature aging and reversed it. (You might want to read my book *How to Be Chic, Fabulous, and Live Forever.*) I considered myself very lucky to be able to do a follow-up on those students that experienced my "visionary healing process"! I have learned now to use these techniques in smaller doses and only in more advanced classes.

The first step to mastering this pattern of excessive family loyalty is to recognize your tendency to copy. If you start getting a disease similar to that of one of your parents, grandparents, or ancestors, you do not have to resign yourself to that disease. Resignation can be deadly. You can rise above the negative thought patterns. You may need the support of knowledgeable and advanced healers who know how to transform the mind and move energy.

The point is that *you can still love your parents without being loyal to all their patterns!*

In my case, I was a rebel, while my sister was a conformist. (She actually died at the same age that my father was when he died.) However, a strange thing happened to me after she died. I began to switch to being a conformist, perhaps to fill the gap somehow for my mother. It felt very strange and did not work for me at all. The whole experience threw me into confusion for a while, and I did not know who I really was. I started to lose my grip. I started to take on my sister's mind, her disease, and whatnot. I also felt guilty that I lived and she did not, and I made up ways to suffer for this guilt. It took me nearly five years to straighten myself out and let those patterns go. It was all an unconscious process, and I found it was amazing as I watched it all play out.

Never underestimate the power of the subconscious mind trickery of the ego. Why do you suppose that the masters strongly recommend that we stay on the spiritual path? We must be alert, for one thing. And we must learn the techniques to handle all the unconscious stuff, for another thing.

I am not a geneticist and I do not want to get into any arguments with geneticists. All I want to point out is this: if someone can materialize his body and dematerialize his body at will, as I have witnessed my guru Babaji do, then there is a lot about the human mind that we don't understand!

If you still think all this is crazy, try reading some of the books written about the ancient teachings of the masters in India. I strongly recommend the series by Robert E. Svoboda titled *Aghora: At the Left Hand of God* and *Aghora II: Kundalini.* I can tell you that it is incredible material and I can hardly digest it. What these writings have taught me is that there is something far beyond modern science. There is the Divine Mother—the Eternal One who is Supreme and the Great Healer. If you are stuck in a family disease, start praying to the Divine Mother!

Addiction to Suffering

I had never noticed I had such an insidious addiction to suffering until recently. That was because when I compared myself to most people, it seemed that I was doing okay. Yes, I had gone through a lot of devastating experiences, and I had experienced many unhealthy conditions in my body, but at least I was not in and out of hospitals, and so on. I felt quite resilient. I felt pleased that I had not become bitter because of the trials of life. I was not depressed or moody; in fact, most of the time I was happy despite my symptoms. I felt so fortunate that I could travel about freely, even though I was not rich. I had just enough money. Therefore, I never counted my symptoms as a form of suffering. I just blamed them on overwork. However, this mistake kept me from facing the area of my mind that I needed to face.

When I got really serious about healing *all* my symptoms, I had to do an in-depth study of myself to learn why I was not letting them go. Then I discovered that because of my religious upbringing, I thought I needed to suffer in some way because the church said suffering is "holy." If I wanted to be holy—and I did—then I could never have the perfect life, free of suffering. "If you suffer now, you get to heaven later," I remember them saying. (What a brainwashing for torture!) So there it was—always making sure I had some symptoms. I would heal one and then just accept another. That way I could also make sure I was not perfect.

As I grew enlightened and happier and happier, it seemed I should somehow suffer even *more* because of the guilt of being happy. (In church, somehow you are not supposed to be too happy.) So it turned out that the happier I grew, the worse my symptoms became, so that I could not stay happy. That was insane! I started resenting the church again—a dangerous attitude, according to church warnings. If you dare to question the church, you will surely suffer—and even more later!

Oh, I was able to function all right. I was able to work and even have a fairly good time . . . but something always kept me from experiencing ecstasy. It seemed to elude me. And that something turned out to be my ego, of course, mainly the part of my ego that was trying to convince me that I had to suffer.

After I recognized this pattern and started to give it up, my mind went into the next phase: a new reason to suffer! Others are suffering; I should be like others if I am to be here and want to be close to them. After all, I could not be the only one around in perfect health! I would be too different. And I was already too different. People might think I was a fake. So I had better suffer somewhat to be accepted, to be considered "normal." This was the next trick of my ego.

On top of all this nonsense, somehow I had it wired up that if I had symptoms like my father and sister, both of whom had died, I would somehow still be connected to them. If I became totally healed, I might want to stay here and then I might not get to go to "heaven" and be with them again. Furthermore, I felt guilty that I was able to live, and that guilt made more symptoms. All this was unconscious, mind you. It is a wonder I did not land in the hospital. I had to stay on top of it constantly for that not to happen. It was work. Fortunately, I had read *A Course in Miracles*, which says, "God's will for us is perfect happiness." This book, which is a correction of religion, helped me straighten out this *mess*.

Then one day in India, while visiting the great saint Shastriji, I noticed that he was always in ecstasy. He never suffered. Besides, he kept shouting to me, "I want you to have intense joy!" Now, try to imagine the effect that had on me. There he was—the living example of what I wanted to be right in front of me. That is what I needed to see, what I needed to hear. And it was *real*. That is why I went to India in the first place: I needed to see examples. In one's spiritual life, such experience is called "The Principle of Right Association"; that is, you associate with that which you want to become. You hang out with those who force you to *adapt upward*.

So I recommend that you become aware of all the forms of suffering you might be creating. One can create suffering anywhere—

in the body, at work, in a relationship, even on vacation. Become committed to giving up suffering. Talk to Jesus about it, to Babaji, to the Divine Mother. Pray about it. This process should also help you become aware of all that you feel guilty about. (See "Guilt and Sickness" on page 53.)

Read *A Course in Miracles* until you unravel false religious theology. There *is* a way out. Keep studying it until you absolutely know that you are innocent and that guilt is not of God.

For meditation, study *A Course in Miracles* lessons: "God's will for me is perfect happiness." "I choose the joy of God instead of pain." "Other people's suffering is not my own."

You may also have to focus forgiveness on the church and your ministers and teachers who misprogrammed you. Forgive yourself for buying it. You knew as a kid that something was really *off* about that, didn't you, really? But we try to please our authority figures. If we challenge them as kids, we usually get put down. If you stood up to them as a kid, good for you. If they put you down for it, forgive that too.

Anger

Anger is very damaging to your etheric substances and organs. It is also damaging to your relationships. When your relationships break down, your body breaks down. *A Course in Miracles* says, "Anger provokes separation, and communication ends separation," as well as, "Anger is never justified."

So what do you do about anger? I have written a lot about this in *Loving Relationships II*. However, some of it is worth repeating here: You should not suppress anger; that is bad for your body. But if you express it, that is bad for others. So you need a way to handle this dilemma. My teacher Babaji gave me the way. He says that you must change the thought that causes the anger and breathe out the energy. Are you willing to do that for the sake of your health?

A lot of people might protest this technique, saying that the anger overtakes them too quickly—before they can change the thought. However, this is a discipline that you can learn if you are willing to try. First notice the feeling of anger coming up. Then immediately start breathing out the heavy energy and try to change the thought coming up. It is really not hard if you put consciousness to it. It helps to have breathwork so you know how to exhale anger and grow used to observing your thoughts and changing them.

For example, you can actually say, "I am feeling angry now about . . ." or "This is my thought that makes me angry ___." Then change it to the opposite and continue. "I am going to run around the block, get breathwork, scream in the shower, whatever."

You change the thought then and there. You do not have to dump the anger on someone else. That is just a bad habit. As you get quicker at this process and learn to change the thought sooner, the anger will actually dissolve right then if you are willing. Besides, it is probably not really *that person* that is making you angry. It is probably someone whom they represent in your past. Furthermore, you might be antagonizing them just to have an excuse to fight. What is your part in provoking this?

I was conducting a marriage consultation once, and the husband told me he did not have to be the one to ask for forgiveness, because she, his wife, started the argument. Therefore it was all her fault. I had to practically go over the whole LRT for him to understand that both cocreated that moment. He could not express any feelings, which caused her to express double feelings. What he suppressed, she expressed. He needed her to do that so he could re-create his childhood and feel what was "familiar." She was, of course, just as responsible. We all cocreate every moment.

Imagine putting a little baby in a pressure cooker that was on all the time. Would you do it? Of course not! So why would you do that to your body? You should always treat your body as kindly as you would a little baby's. I don't even let my body stay in the space of other people's anger. If anyone starts yelling and screaming, I leave. I am too sensitive. Of course, I look at my part in any dilemma, but I can look at my part of that outside the room and still protect my body. After all, we do have free will to put our bodies where we want.

I hope that now I am at peace enough so that all people around me feel that peace and want to be at peace in my presence. (That does not mean there is no excitement.) People who can maintain high levels of love and excitement and ecstasy without quickly blowing up afterward are getting somewhere. That probably means their subconscious is clear of anger. They can maintain peace in high energy. High energy tends to bring up anything unlike itself. You can tell a lot about people by watching them in high energy situations, especially afterward. They might go nuts for days afterward. It is absolutely not true that you cannot control your anger. Who *is* in control of it? Of course you are. To think that you are not is a cop-out.

Here is what some gurus say on the subject:

Guru Mai:

> *It is said that if you are a true ascetic, you are completely devoid of anger. If there is any trace of anger in you, you are called a scoundrel, not an ascetic. A great being will go to any extent to remove the fire of anger. The greatness of a Saddhu Monk is that he can drop something once he realizes he has it.*

Dalai Lama:

> *We lose control of our mind through hatred and anger. If our minds are dominated by anger, we will lose the best part of human intelligence—wisdom! Anger is one of the most serious problems facing the world today. ("A Human Approach to World Peace" a pamphlet, page 12)*

Mata Amritanandamayi (The Mother):

> *Anger and impatience will always cause problems. Suppose you have a weakness of getting angry easily. Once you become normal again, go and sit in the family shrine room or in solitude and regret and repent your anger. Sincerely pray to your beloved deity or Mother Nature, seeking help to get rid of it. TRY TO MAKE YOUR OWN MIND AWARE OF THE BAD OUTCOME OF ANGER. When you are angry at someone, you lose all your mental balance. Your discriminative power completely stops functioning. You say whatever comes into your mind and act accordingly. You may even utter crude words.*
>
> *By acting and thinking with anger, you lose a lot of good energy. Become aware that these negative feelings will only pave the way for your own destruction! (Awaken Children, pages 4–5)*

Amma also says anger makes you weak in every pore of your body.

What to Do During an Anger Attack

1. Do not yell at anyone else.

2. Lie down and breathe, pumping out your anger on the exhale. (It helps to know how to do conscious breathwork.)

3. If that does not work, run around the block until calm.

4. When you calm down, remind yourself of these two lines from *A Course in Miracles*:

   A. "You will attack what does not satisfy you to avoid seeing that you created it."

   B. "Beware of the temptation to perceive yourself as unjustly treated."

5. This means you created the result at which you are angry. You somehow wanted it, needed it, or are addicted to it, so try to get enlightened about this fact and see your part! (What is your payoff? What are you getting out of this that is neurotic?)

6. Express yourself sanely now.

   A. "I felt angry because . . ."

   B. "I see now that I had the thought . . . that attracted this situation."

   C. "I apologize for this and I want to repent and make amends."

7. Do the process recommended by the Mother, Mata Amritanandamayi, in a holy area.

8. If you are not completely calm, write down all your feelings of anger and then burn the paper.

9. If the above does not work, you need more help. Call a friend who is more enlightened than you at the time to get help "processing."

10. Do a Truth Process such as "The reason I do not want to forgive is . . ." (Usually seeing your part in the situation dilutes the problem quite a bit if you are telling the truth.)

continued on next page

11. Remember that forgiveness is the key to happiness and health.

12. Remember that behind every grievance, there is a miracle.

13. Remember that anger is one of the causes of aging and death. (It is *not* worth it.)

14. Follow Catherine Ponder's steps to forgiveness:
    A. You forgive them.
    B. You forgive yourself.
    C. Allow them to forgive you.
    D. Give up all desire to punish and get even.
    E. Restore good harmony as before the upset.

Guilt and Sickness

Guilt demands punishment—that is, in your ego mind, you believe that is so. One of the ways we punish ourselves when we feel guilty is to get sick. We attack our bodies with an illness, pain, or injury that we actually make up.

A Course in Miracles says that guilt is not only not of God, it is actually an attack on God! It says it is a sure sign that your thinking is unnatural. This is all explained in a section called "The Ego's Use of Guilt." *A Course* also says that if you have guilt, you are walking the carpet of death. (That means that we think we must eventually die as a form of punishment for our guilt, especially since we think we are such sinners! We therefore kill ourselves with our own thoughts, squeezing the life force right out of ourselves.)

Sometimes, however, you may not even realize you are guilty until you get a symptom. In this way, the symptoms serve you to make you aware of the guilt. A few years back, I developed a lot of tension as a result of having to fire someone. It is the part of my job as a leader that I hate the most. I figured out that the tension was due to the guilt, but I could not seem to shake it. So I discussed it with someone more spiritually advanced at that moment. That teacher gave me some real feedback. He said, "Your problem as a leader is that you don't ever let people fall on their faces." He made it clear to me that some people set it up that way to finally learn their lessons. In effect, they "fire" themselves! I appreciated that teaching, and I did not let his criticism of me incur more guilt and tension. I welcome criticism, especially when I need it. So the moral of the story is that if you cannot get rid of your guilt, get spiritual help before you destroy your body.

Reading *A Course in Miracles* also helps you become regrounded in your innocence. It says you can have forgiveness in the "Holy Instant" because God does not make your sins real. (*Sins* means your "case," your "mistakes.") That is because God knows that your "case" is just your ego, which is not real. This may seem like an advanced concept if you have not read all of *A Course in Miracles.* Another way to say this is, "Your ego is a nightmare that you are temporarily experiencing." You think you are separate (ego), but that is not real. (When your child has a nightmare, for example, you don't make *it* real, nor does God make our nightmares real.) It is important to keep studying *CIM (A Course in Miracles)* until you finally understand this point.

Along with the idea of guilt, one must beware of the danger of carrying "deep dark secrets." This is like having inside you a festering boil full of guilt, which you pretend you do not have and it does not affect your body! This keeps eating away at you . . . no doubt about it. You must be willing to tell someone if you have some deep secret about which you feel guilty. That was one of the whole ideas of going to a priest. However, confession has in many cases been used to make one feel even more guilty. It might be better to share your dark secret with someone you really trust. Get it off your chest.

An acquaintance of mine was killed in a small plane crash. I had a lot of trouble understanding why he had crashed, because he was quite enlightened; I wanted to know what went wrong with his mind to attract that fate. I begged one of my teachers (who is a seer) to tell me. He was reluctant, but after he saw the insomnia I suffered because of that death, he said that this man had a deep, dark secret. I later found out that he was in fact a very secretive person. In the end, this did him in because he never released all his guilt. He tried to hide it.

So I started teaching my students to confess their deep secrets. One girl finally told the whole group her father was in the Mafia! Her whole life changed after that. She became younger and very powerful in her own right.

Once I did something I thought was really stupid, and I could not let go of it. One friend knew about it, but it was still not enough for me to tell just him. He realized I needed some kind of ceremony. So he put me in his car and drove me out in the woods to meet a friend of his, an actual recluse. He told me to go into the shack and confess this thing to his friend, the recluse. Well, I did it. I have no idea who that recluse was or is to this day, but he was very loving. He did not know who I was either, and he did not care. He just heard what I said and loved me and did not bat an eye. He thought it was trivial. I obviously got over the whole thing by confessing, because I cannot even remember what it was about now.

Years later I found myself with a very silly habit that I was really embarrassed about. I could not seem to overcome it for a whole year; and because I was a public figure, I did not want to tell anyone. It was too embarrassing. But then I remembered the friend who had driven me to see the recluse, so I went to see the same man who took me to the recluse. He was hanging out in the kitchen with another wild friend in San Diego. Now, this guy was the opposite of a recluse. He was rich and all that, and he was "cool." I decided this was the moment and I had to do it; I blurted out my bad habit. I was so embarrassed. They looked at me, and they both said in unison, "So what?" Then they went right on to something else a lot more interesting! The next day I was cured. The habit disappeared from my life forever.

Find a stranger if you don't have anyone else to talk to. Try it!

Fear and Sickness

This chapter is my own summary from a year of studying *A Course in Miracles.*

A Course in Miracles says all healing is essentially the release from fear. It also says only two true emotions exist: love and fear. Love is God. That won't make you sick. Fear is ego. That *will* make you sick.

Fear may seem beyond your control, but it is not. Fear is self-controlled. We *are* responsible for what we think. When we have fear, *CIM* says, it is a sure sign we have allowed our minds to miscreate. When we are fearful, we have chosen wrongly. The correction of fear, then, is *our* responsibility. When we ask God to take away our fear, we imply that it is not our responsibility. We must ask instead for help with the conditions that have brought our fears about. A condition that produces fear, according to *CIM*, is our desire to remain separate from God. Our fear presents us from letting the Holy Spirit be in charge. If we let the Holy Spirit be in charge, no fear will exist. Fear is, then, a result of our "control number."

A Course says that attempting to master fear is useless because that gives fear more power. The only way to overcome fear is to master love. Fear comes from thoughts. By choosing loving thoughts, you are rejecting fear. In *CIM*, Jesus offers these steps to the release of fear:

1. Know first that this is fear.
2. Fear arises from lack of love.
3. The only remedy for lack of love is perfect love.
4. Perfect love is the Atonement.

In *CIM*, the Atonement means allowing the Holy Spirit to correct all your wrong thinking.

This is a really powerful quotation from *CIM:* "*I (Jesus) know it (fear) does not exist; but you do not. You believe in the power of what does not exist.*"

What He is saying is that fear does not really exist, because fear is the ego and the ego is separation; the separation does not exist. But we have made the separation seem to be real, and therefore, we have made the ego seem to be real. Therefore, we have made fear seem real. If we, in fact, think we are separate from God, we will have fear.

Anytime we are sick, we replace God with the ego. The part of our body that suffers is where we are storing our ego and pushing out God. That is why *CIM* says that "sickness is idolatry." It actually goes so far as to say that when you are sick, you are trying to kill God!

The body cannot act wrongly unless it is responding to mis-thoughts. It is your thoughts alone that cause you pain and sickness. It is a fundamental error to think that the body creates. *A Course* will tell you this over and over: that if you are sick, you are withdrawing from God. You are spiritually deprived. It will tell you over and over that all forms of illness are physical expressions of fear.

There is the fear that causes sickness, and then there is the fear of healing on top of that. The reason healing is a threat is that it would mean that you *are* responsible for your thoughts. In other words, the mind makes the decision to be sick and all illness is mental illness. People often do not want to face this fact. They would rather blame something outside themselves. It seems easier. However, if you keep doing that, how can you ever heal yourself?

People are often afraid of healing, because if they have chosen sickness as a way of life to get attention, they might lose that attention and get really depressed.

People are often very afraid of the miracle healings they say they want. They may pray for a miracle, but they are actually terrified of miracles. That is because experiencing a miracle would change their whole reality. The thought of accepting a miracle is terrifying to most people. So *CIM* recommends that you clearly understand how to pray for healing. It recommends that you do not pray for a miracle healing of your cancer or arthritis to happen overnight. You have too much fear of that much light, of that much reality shifting that fast. You most likely would not let it happen unless you were in the presence of Jesus Himself or Mary at the shrine, where you would feel completely safe.

In *CIM*, Jesus says to pray for the *removal of the* fear *of healing* first. After all, the Holy Spirit is not going to *add* to your fear! If you are terrified of miracles, he is not going to scare the hell out of you with one. You must prepare your mind. You must be ready for miracles. You must be over the fear of healing before you will let it happen.

It took me a long, long time to understand these points in the *CIM*. When I finally integrated this information, I was able to adjust the techniques that I explain later in this book. In other words, if you are not giving up a condition, you must find out why you *fear* giving up that condition. (Don't worry; this will all become clearer to you later.)

Misery, pain, suffering, and death—we are all used to them. We are also addicted to them (ego). What we are really afraid of is life, God, and love. So this makes us hang onto conditions that bring us down in energy—to a state that is more familiar than all the energy we would have in a state of absolute pristine and perfect health or in the incredible light-energy of a miracle.

We are so confused that we actually think God kills people. If God is energy, then in that way of thinking, energy kills people. So we are also terrified of energy. And yet the truth is, the energy of God can heal you completely. But you must get your mind straight first or you will stop the whole process.

The Atonement cures all sickness, Jesus said. The Atonement takes away guilt. Your cure comes from your holiness.

Suppressing fear causes pain. Feel the fear, breathe it out, and change the thoughts that cause it. It is the same treatment I gave you for anger. Ask for correction of the *cause* of your fear and your fearful thoughts. The cause is the belief in separation. The only thing you need to correct is your *imagined* separation.

You may need to read this section several times. I wrote it in ten minutes with the "Ave Maria" turned up very loud so I would not be blocked and my own mind would not get in the way.

The Unconscious Death Urge

One of the *main* causes of sickness and symptoms is what we call the unconscious death urge. This is the ego in its worst form. It includes the following:

The thought "I am separate from God"

The belief that "death is inevitable"

All your programming from society and family about death

Your family patterns on disease, aging, and death

The invalidation of your personal divinity

Addictions and bad habits leading to aging and death

Any antilife thoughts

Your secret wish to die because you hate your life

False religious theology

Past-life memories of dying

All of this is like a *conglomerate* in your subconscious mind. It will run you until you take charge of your mind and clear it. This can be done. In every religious tradition, there are great Immortals who overcome death. (See the "Physical Immortality" chapter on page 79.)

If you constantly affirm "death is inevitable," death is the result you will get. The way to create death is to create aging and sickness so you can die. In the Bible, Jesus actually said, "The power of life and death are in the tongue." That, of course, means that what you *say* is what you *get* in your body. You are at cause over your body. Your body is like a computer printout; you are the programmer!

Most people believe that death is beyond their control. Some blame it on God. But if you believe that God controls your death, you are making God a murderer! Others blame something out there in the universe, as if "something" is out to get them. If that is the case, it is impossible to walk around in the universe and relax. Your physical body will break down with all this tension of wondering when "it" is going to get you. Besides, if you try to live while having the thought that "death is inevitable," it is like trying to drive a car forward at 90 mph with the gears in reverse. It strips the gears and the car breaks down. Your body will break down. Of course, you can also use accidents as a way to kill yourself.

Your physical body is obviously your most valuable possession. However, have you noticed that people take better care of their cars and houses than they do their own bodies? People allow their bodies to be destroyed, sometimes easily, without protest.

Actually, your *mind* kills your body. Therefore, all death is suicide! *A Course in Miracles* says, "Death is a result of a thought called the Ego." People use their egos to kill themselves. If you believe that death is inevitable, you are in the process of dying right now. You are programming it right now. If you heal one disease and do not change that thought, you will just make up another one to kill yourself. That is why Leonard Orr said, "All healing is temporary until you heal death." What is the point of learning to heal yourself, then, if you will just keep trying to kill yourself?

The minute we forgot who we were and created the fall (separation-ego), death was invented as our own punishment for that "sin." The belief in sin is the self-command for punishment and death. Once you accept the idea that you are separate from God, it is all downhill after that. Then you will have thoughts such as, "I don't have any power. I am weak. I cannot heal myself. I don't deserve life."

Our society is raised in "deathist" mentality. We are hypnotized by the thought that death is inevitable. This belief system is like many belief systems—something we were taught. We think belief systems make us feel safe, even if they are killing us! This is a false sense of safety. Are you willing to change a belief system? When you get outside belief systems, you start experiencing mastery. You go to *direct knowing*. And that is thrilling.

Most people cannot imagine wanting to live forever and giving up their death urge, because they are in so much pain. What they do not realize is that the reason they are in pain in the first place is because of their death urge. Catch-22. One must figure out this.

Your death urge could be operating in many areas of your life. The obvious one is your body. However, you might also be "killing off" your relationships, your business, your friendships, and whatnot. You may be losing money in investments because you are killing them off. Never underestimate the power of the ego and the death urge.

Later in this book I present more information showing how to use the knowledge of Physical Immortality as a healing force in your body and life. For now, it is important to see that the death urge causes disease, not the other way around. People think they get sick, age, and then die. What they really do is die in their minds, which causes sickness and aging.

One main point of *A Course in Miracles* is that hell is what the ego makes of the present. We create our own hells with our ego, and then, after misusing our power and creating hell, we think we deserve to die. In our minds, death becomes the only way out. And according to our egos, we don't think we deserve to live even if we wanted to! Usually we don't want to live because we turned our life into hell: pain, misery, suffering, and aging. *A Course* spends a long time showing you your "descent into hell." To get out of all this, you must become a master . . . but that was the whole point of your life in the first place!

Past Lives and Sickness

I was not aware of the effects of past lives when I was young. I did not even know about the subject! It was certainly not something ever discussed in church (even though I have now found references in the Bible about masters who lived "before" as someone else). And this topic was certainly not something discussed in medicine when I studied nursing.

When I finally made it to California in the '70s, I was, of course, compelled to read books such as Edgar Cayce's that really opened me up to past-life ideas. And after breathwork started, I had to look at the subject more closely. One day I had a client who began remembering being in a war in Ireland. She suddenly began speaking with a perfect Irish accent during the session. She certainly was not Irish in this life—that was obvious. Later I asked her if she had ever been to Ireland and she said no. I asked her if she had ever studied the Irish dialect and she said no. I asked her if she remembered speaking to me in long paragraphs with an Irish accent without hesitation. She was able to remember the scenes, but the speaking only vaguely.

Also, some time after that, I began to have more and more past-life memories in my own breathwork sessions. I saw scenes that were clearly from other eras and nothing that I had ever glimpsed in any movie, either. The styles of furniture and architecture were very different from anything I had known in my current life. The main thing that always amazed me was that I had such strong emotions while having those memories. They were so spontaneous and real to me that I knew I could not be making that up. It was too strong. Why would I want to make that up anyway? I started paying attention.

Then I went to India for the first time. It was after that visit that I began to have past-life memories frequently. It was as if my guru Babaji was deliberately pushing them into my mind to be cleared. There was no way I could avoid this clearing, whether I liked it or not. And it has been going on for years and years now. Recently, the much more difficult ones have come up.

Now I can relate to many stories told by clients with illnesses they couldn't seem to heal until they came to us for breathwork. Quite frankly, I can say that breathwork with a past-life regression did the trick. I am very happy that this kind of healing is now being adequately and professionally researched. I would definitely refer everyone to the book *Other Lives, Other Selves* by Dr. Roger Woolger (Bantam Books, 1988). I called him personally immediately after reading it. This book is a must for all breathworkers and healers, and I also recommend it to all clients. It is hard to put down. I think it must have made a huge impact on the field of psychology by now. In the first chapter, Dr. Woolger acknowledges that he was a skeptic who encountered past lives only when he started breathwork. The professional studies he has done are truly awesome.

On page 100, Dr. Woolger states:

> *The body and its various aches, pains and dysfunctions is a living psychic history when read correctly. Even though the physical ailment may have very specific origins in a person's current life, I have found more and more that there are certain layers to every major syndrome of physical illness, accident, or weakness. The existence of a past life level of physical problems has been confirmed over and over again in the cases I have seen.*

On page 101:

> *A woman in her early forties relived an unfulfilled life as a woman in the pioneer days which ended tragically when a horse and trap overturned; she broke her back and died when she was twenty-seven in that life. In this life, at age twenty-seven, she was in the hospital with a very serious kidney infection which they could not properly diagnose and she nearly died. . . . The pain was absolutely terrible and was in the same place where she had broken her back in the other life.*

On page 143, he describes his work with phobias:

Although many phobias do, indeed, arise in this life, it seems to be the case that almost everyone has some particular deep fear that will not be thus explained. Whether it be fear of spiders, wild animals, fire, water, heights, crowds, knives, dark places, and so on. I have consistently found that behind that fear lies a specific and detailed story of a past-life trauma. In sessions, people remember deaths from poisonous insects, from spiders, snakes, sharks, and more. Many who fear heights recall deaths from being thrown off cliffs, falling from planes in recent wars, etc.

"Increasingly," he says (page 171), "in practicing psychotherapy from a past-life perspective, I am convinced that the likelihood of cure depends on whether or not I am able to guide my client to the crucial or key story from his or her past lives. My experience indicates that if we can reach such a story in the early session, cure will be correspondingly swift."

This book also contains stories about how gynecological problems related to past lives of sexual abuse and rape. There are many detailed accounts about how these ancient traumas relate to present-day frigidity and lack of orgasm in women.

PART III

Framework for Healing

Your Relationship with Your Symptoms

When you develop symptoms or a disease, you might react to the situation in a number of different ways:

You might deny it is going on at all.

You might acknowledge it but avoid it.

You might be angry at the situation.

You might even fight it and get in a battle with your mind.

You might resist it.

You might hate yourself for it.

You might continually complain about it.

You might continually worry about it.

You might even get obsessed with it.

You might get really depressed about it.

You might overdose with food, liquor, or drugs to suppress it.

You might get terrified of it.

You might mistakenly think it has more power than you do.

It is extremely tempting to take one of these approaches, especially if the symptoms stick around. The trouble is that "what you resist persists," so these approaches only fortify the symptoms. Remember the metaphysical principle that "what you think about expands"! So the more you dwell on it in a negative way, the worse it will get. True, it *is* hard not to dwell on it negatively, especially when it is painful. But it will get even more painful when you dwell on it. Denying it is not good either. You need to learn from it and take the necessary action to change.

So then you really must get a hold of your mind. *A Course in Miracles* says that "the physician is the mind of the patient himself." This means you are your own doctor: you created the symptom and you can uncreate it. But you must start by giving up the above tempting tendencies, and you must develop a loving relationship with your symptom or disease. How do you do that? Ah, yes, that is the trick!

First, acknowledge it as a blessing . . . in that it is there to show you that your mind is *off.* It is there to teach you something very important. It is there to teach you that your mind needs correction. It is there to get your attention.

Second, ask the symptom, "What are you trying to tell me?" Or have a friend ask you the question, "If your symptom could talk, what would it say to you?" The answer is within. It is not acceptable to say "I don't know." You *do* know. The answer is within. Your partner or friend should not accept that answer. They must then say to you, "If you did know, what would it be?"/"I don't know" comes from not looking. For exact information on the cause of this condition, do the Ultimate Truth Process from this book (page 97). This is a very, very important step in self-analysis. If you want *Permanent Healing,* you must know the *cause.*

Third, try the techniques in this book. If the symptom or disease does not shift after self-analysis (the Truth Process and breathwork, for example), you need much more understanding of the framework in this book and the techniques given later. You should go to a breathworker, for example, and find out why you do not want to be healed.

Fourth, remember that the sickness is the "cure in process." This means you take the attitude of experiencing your condition as a purging of negative thought or construct, rather than as something stuck. Taking this attitude is very important—it's the basis for your healing. You must train yourself to remember this: Your body is trying to "spit out" the effects of the negative thoughts that caused it. Your body is attempting to cure itself when you have symptoms. You need to mentally cooperate with this healing process. If you fight it, ignore it, or react in one or more of the negative ways mentioned at the beginning of this chapter, you will only add negative mental mass.

Attitude and Frame of Mind

In my opinion, the hardest part of being sick (besides feeling terrible, of course) is the worry that the condition will never end. So often one is tempted to think, "What if I *never* get over this?" This fear can escalate to the point that you actually start thinking you will definitely never get over it. At that point, you may even start feeling like your body controls you instead of you controlling it.

When you have overwhelming fear, you forget that you control your body with your mind and you start thinking that your body or disease controls you—that it is more powerful than you. Then the situation gets even worse because you feel helpless. You are losing it now, and you must take drastic action to realize that *you* are in charge. Your body is never the cause. You are. Your mind is. If you don't correct your mind at this point, you might become paralyzed with fear to the point that the body's automatic healing system literally shuts down. Or you could end up crystallizing the symptoms into something very solid. Therefore, it is really important to get through this danger by having the thought *"This will pass . . ."*

A person may go from doctor to doctor or from healer to healer while none of them can help—because part of the person's mind is trying to prove the condition cannot be healed. That way the person can continue to hate God for his or her plight and remain angry rather than changing. Of course, people who "need" their anger rarely admit it. It is their little secret. Or, they could be in total denial about their war against God. If one were healed and remained healed, felt fantastic, and everything was working, what would there be to get angry at? Some people just do not want to give up their need to blame.

If you create the sickness or symptoms because you want attention, you may not want to be healed either, because you would lose
all the attention. This is another trap! If you create the symptom as
a way of suffering because you believe that you *must* suffer, you
might also set yourself up not to be healed. If you create the sickness or symptoms as a way of punishing yourself for something, you
will probably set yourself up not to be healed because you still think
you need more punishment.

When you finally see no more value in the pain, suffering, and
self-punishment, you will spontaneously heal yourself or finally
manifest the right doctor or healer to help you do the trick. "The
outcome is what the patient decides." It will spontaneously become
obvious what you need to do or where you need to go or with
whom you need to be to end your ailment. "God is ready when you
are." You will probably wonder why it took you so long to recognize
the obvious!

Someone said, "You will be sick until you are sick of being sick."
Or you will get off it when you are *ready* to get off it. One day you
decide this attention you enjoy from the illness is not worth it. Or
you decide you have had enough of an excuse for a break. Or you
decide you no longer have any more fear of being in your full power.
Or you finally forgive. Or whatever.

Many times students who have already taken my spiritual healing class come to me and complain about some ailment they have
had for a long time. I ask them, "Well, what did you get when you
did the Ultimate Truth Process?" Then they confess to me that they
did not do it!

I ask, "Why not?"

"Oh! I *forgot*," they say.

I was always so surprised at this answer at first. But now I understand how tricky the ego is. It distracts you from what works. You
must train yourself to do the Truth Process as soon as you get the
symptoms so they won't escalate. Of course, if you like to suffer or
punish yourself, you won't do the Process even if you do remember.
Sometimes people "forget" because of a deep unconscious fear of
going against the church that told them they must suffer. That distorts
their thinking. In that case, the person needs to be helped by someone
like me or someone else who is no longer trapped in that dogma.

The Ultimate Truth Process is on page 97.

Finding the Solution

Important Points

1. The part of the mind that is *real*, of the Holy Spirit's mind, totally alive and perfect, is *always* there and is always stronger than any mistaken thought of your ego. Your ego miscreated the negative condition.

   Say, "I am stronger than this . . ." or "The God in me is stronger than . . ."

2. Remember again that anything you have created, you can uncreate. It is *actually less work* to heal yourself than to make yourself sick. It takes a lot of effort and struggle to hang onto a lot of negative thinking to make yourself sick. You natural state is health. You had to really work at going against your natural state to have created this condition.

3. Anything on its way up is on its way *out*. That is another way of saying that your symptom is the cure in process. At least it is no longer suppressed!

4. You may need to get a breathworker sooner than you think—one who knows how to "process" or clean your resistance to healing. The breathworker should be able to help you get to the cause of the condition, help you breathe it out, and help you process it yourself if the healing does not work because you are blocking it.

5. The *will to live* is the most important factor in your healing. If your life urge is strong enough, you can definitely overcome. If you get stuck in fear, or "I might die," you will weaken

greatly and inhibit the natural healing abilities of the body. Recently I read an article about a man who had severe metastasis of cancer. He reversed it all and came out clean, much to the shock of doctors who could hardly accept his healing. The one thing I remember about the article is that he said he *never* entertained the thought that he was going to die. Somehow he was able to have absolute certainty—and it worked.

On a plane the other day, I read about the longest living AIDS patient who has beat all odds. What I remember about the article is that he used that very same thinking. He decided, and told his mate, that he was not going to die from it. Doctors keep researching this guy to see why he has beaten the odds. But in the research, they forget to study that very point! They studied his diet, his habits, his relationships, his living style—everything. The conclusion: maybe he is still alive because he meditates. They never mentioned his absolute decision to live. I read about that decision in a different section of the article in which he was discussing that himself.

6. Remember: *Faith is everything!* When your faith is weak and the temptation to think that you won't make it takes over, that is exactly when you need to pray more, get breathwork, and get support.

Spiritual Background

A Course in Miracles *in Review*

A Course in Miracles is a correction of religion. It is important to understand how false religious theology ruins and runs our lives. It is important to understand how it affects our minds, our bodies, and our health. Naturally, much of what we learned in church was wonderful; however, some teachings were intolerably confusing. Until those points are cleared up, it is hard to figure out *Permanent Healing.*

For example, the church teaches that we are separate from God. This mistaken theology leads us to believe that we must die to be with God; therefore, we, of course, get sick and age. We think we are bad for being here because we "left" God to get here. Therefore, we are sinners of the worst kind. If we believe this premise, we will have tremendous guilt—and guilt demands punishment. One of the main ways we punish ourselves is by damaging our bodies, getting sick, aging, and finally choosing death as the final punishment. *A Course* calls this our descent into hell while here on earth.

The church teaches that heaven is somewhere else and is our goal. Therefore, we cannot really wait to leave here, and as a result, we are not fully here. The worst part is that by making statements such as "The Lord took him away" when someone dies, the church teaches that God kills people. This insanity makes us fear and hate God for taking away our loved ones and for making us feel that God does not permit us to live as long as we would like. The church has implied that we should not have too much fun or joy. We are supposed to suffer, so we become addicted to having disease.

Therefore, the joy of having *Permanent Healing* is something we think we do not deserve. Confusion after confusion reigns. These confusions leave us tied up in knots. We supposedly are not even allowed to question the church or we might go to hell. How, then, can one get anything straight? This is exactly why we need *A Course in Miracles*—to straighten things out.

CIM is not a religion or a path. It is a correction. When you read it, you will know it came from Jesus and there is only one appropriate response: gratitude to Him. The reason it is Christian in tone is because Christianity must be corrected first since it is such a major influence on the planet. No body of knowledge exists that does not need to be corrected and upgraded. However, many religions are threatened by the ideas in *CIM*, because it challenges what is false. Some do not want to change even though they profess that they do not like the horrors afflicting society and that something must be done. Before anyone criticizes *CIM*, I should think they need to read it all the way through. This is common sense. If adverse critics would read it all the way through before criticizing it, I think they would change their tune.

A Course in Miracles explains that everything we know is wrong, so we must start over. (Our results should show us that.) Everything is wrong because we interpret everything through the ego. The ego is a false self that we made up to compete with God. It is based on the erroneous thought "I am separate from God." Once we believed that, we went into weakness, helplessness, fear, anxiety, suffering, anger, misery, sickness, aging, and death.

In the ego's interpretation, this separation is real and actually happened. Therefore, God is out to destroy us for this. So we try to bargain with God, saying, "You don't have to go to the trouble of punishing me; I will punish myself." The idea of sacrifice was then formed: "I will suffer and deprive myself to prove I am good, so you won't be angry, God." In the ego's thought system, we get the insane notion that sacrifice is salvation, that God's will for us is perfect misery, and that we do not deserve to be happy. Furthermore, we think that the more we suffer now, the better off we will be later on (such as in heaven).

The ego's version is that we must perish. (I acknowledge the great teacher Ken Wapnick, one of the leading experts on *CIM*, for helping me understand it.)

The ego's interpretation of the crucifixion is that only one of God's sons (Jesus) had to suffer to free us all. However, this interpretation lays more guilt on our heads; that is, how does it make you feel if someone who is totally pure must die for you? This interpretation, Ken explained, does not make us feel free of guilt at all; yet salvation is supposed to free us from guilt. Obviously, we do not really understand the crucifixion. This is again why we need *A Course in Miracles.* It explains that the crucifixion was an extreme teaching device. It shows that no perception of oneself as a victim is justified. It explains that Jesus did not defend himself, nor did he even believe he was attacked. He saw only threatened people who did not think they deserved the love of God.

In *CIM*, Jesus says that the truth is that there is no sin because there is no separation. The truth is that it is impossible for us to separate from God. Therefore, we are innocent. All sins are forgiven because they never really occurred. So there is no need for sacrifice. Because you are innocent, you do not need to suffer, and because that is true, you can also give yourself perfect health now!

Personally, it has taken me a long time to digest *CIM* because I was addicted to the dogma of the church for so many lifetimes. I, like most people, brought to this life certain core beliefs that seemed impossible to change—such as "We are sinners." It seemed that if I gave up the thought that I am a sinner, I would *really* be a sinner. Or if I dared think I was innocent, I would *really* be guilty. This is the *trap* of the ego. What helped me most was to remember this: if there is a lie at the center of a thought system, the whole system is deceptive. Since the lie at the center of my religion was that one is separate from God, I had to admit that the whole religion is off. Even after I understood that, I was still afraid because the church had an extra, built-in control number: if I questioned that, or tried to leave, I would surely die and go to hell.

But one day I realized all this was really ridiculous because on the one hand, they used the threat of death to control me, and on the other hand, they promoted death as something to look forward to for final peace! This double bind was not resolvable, and so I knew it had to be off. I resented being put into this trap my whole life. I regretted buying into it. Through prayer and help from my teachers, I have been able to unravel this conflict to the point that things make more sense. I know now that many of the illnesses I have manifested and mentioned in this book were a direct result of this religious brainwashing and confusion. (Some people now call it religious abuse.)

I do not want to be on a campaign to attack religion. I have tried to forgive all false religious theology. What I want is to be able to understand what is false and what is real—and Jesus is telling us *now*. He says the Holy Spirit was placed in our minds as a solution to our imagined separation. To Jesus, our identity is spirit. Therefore, we are love, joy, happiness, bliss, peace, and perfect health. There is even the possibility of immortality if one follows his words and practices spiritual laws. He even said this in the Bible: "If you follow me, you will never see the grave." Few could do it; however, some did and became Immortal masters who ascended (dematerialized).

Often when Immortals try to explain that giving up the death urge is the key to having perfect health and that Physical Immortality is a real possibility, others cannot accept such information because their minds are in the other framework (ego). So it is like talking to a wall or speaking in a foreign language. To understand the idea of *Permanent Healing*, one must have one's mind in the opposite framework. One literally must know the difference between the ego's thought system and the Holy Spirit's thought system. (And this is not Freud's definition of the ego.) People in the ego's thought system think that death is inevitable—and it will be. They think death is the will of God.

I have chosen only two paragraphs to quote from *A Course in Miracles*. If you read them carefully, I think you will be stunned. However, the rest of *CIM* is just as astounding. Imagine your awe if you should read the whole *Course*!

The problem is that the ego tries to keep us from learning that which would heal us. So there may be tremendous resistance even to buying *CIM*. There could be more resistance to reading it. The books say that *CIM* is required if you want to make it—only the time you take is voluntary. This means you can get it in the next five months, the next five years, or the next five lifetimes. But why wait? Why not now?

Read the following, substituting the word *sickness*. All sickness and symptoms are part of the death urge and ego. Sickness and death are correlative.

Death is not your Father's will nor yours. The death
penalty is the ego's ultimate goal, for it truly believes
that you are a criminal deserving death. The death
penalty never leaves the ego's mind, for that is what it
always reserves for you in the end. It will torment you
while you live, but its hatred is not satisfied until you
die. As long as you feel guilty, you are listening to the
voice of the ego, which tells you that you have been
treacherous to God and therefore deserve death.

Try to stay with this. Read it as many times as you need to. It
could be the key to your healing and health.

You will think that death comes from God and not from
the ego, because by confusing yourself with the ego, you
think you want death. When you are tempted by the
desire for death, remember that I DID NOT DIE. (Jesus
speaking.) Would I have overcome death for myself
alone? And would eternal life be given to one of the
Father's sons, unless He had also given it to you?

When you learn to make ME manifest, you will never
see death. God did not make death. But if you use the
world for what is not its purpose, you will not escape
the laws of disease, violence and death. FORGET NOT
THAT THE HEALING OF GOD'S SONS (ALL SOULS)
IS ALL THE WORLD IS FOR.

"No one can die unless he chooses death." What seems to be the
fear of death is really its attraction.

When you make sin real, you request death. To the ego, sin
means death, so Atonement is achieved through murder!

DEATH IS THE RESULT OF THE THOUGHT WE
CALL THE EGO, JUST AS SURELY AS LIFE IS THE
RESULT OF THE THOUGHT WE CALL GOD.

Death is an attempt to resolve conflict by not deciding
at all. Like any other solution the ego attempts, it will
not work. To the ego, the goal is death. The ego is
insane.

A Course says hell is what the ego makes of the *present*. The way out of our own hell is to accept the Atonement for ourselves. That means inviting in the Holy Spirit and accepting the correction of all our wrong thinking. It means not giving support or agreement to anyone else's illusions of sickness and death. It means having the right perception of the body.

> *When the body becomes an empty space, without any*
> *purpose other than the one the Holy Spirit gives it, it*
> *can become a sign of life, a promise of redemption, a*
> *breath of immortality to those grown sick of breathing*
> *in the fetid scent of death. The Will of God, who created*
> *neither sin nor death, wills that you not be bound by*
> *them.*

Jesus goes on to say in *CIM* that nothing is accomplished through death. Everything is accomplished through life, and life is of the mind and in the mind. He says that if we share the same mind, we can overcome death, because he did.

Physical Immortality

If you have the ability to destroy your body (which takes a whole lot of effort), you can just as well preserve it, which is a great deal easier. However, if you believe death is inevitable and that you are separate from God, you are in the process of dying right now.

"Oh," you might say, "a hundred years of this is all I can take." This statement springs from a deep-rooted belief in suffering and limitation. You have not yet experienced the fullness of health, joy, wisdom, peace, and love. You are given the means by which to have these substantive qualities of life itself; and once you have them, why leave?

The corollary of death is sickness. By the way, *A Course in Miracles* says that sickness is idolatry!

Some people say, "Well, I am willing to live forever if it does not get too bad." That is a cop-out because it only gets too bad if one has not given up loyalty to death. In other words, the reason one has pain, suffering, misery, and a bad time is precisely because of hanging onto the death urge.

People think that you age, you get sick, and you die. The truth is, "You die in your mind, you get sick, and then you age." You create symptoms in your body that make it socially acceptable to leave it.

Your beliefs control your physical body. If you think you are going to die, you will. However, death is *optional*. And there is also an alternative to aging! The key to that is to stop affirming that "death is inevitable." This will definitely improve your health.

Choosing life strengthens your body the most. That means choosing life so fully that you love it so much you want to live forever. *That kind of passion is what works.* Physical Immortality can be defined as *"endless existence,"* specifically the endless existence of your physical body in perpetual health and youthfulness. The body may look different . . . we must learn about that. It would be a "Diamond Body." (See "The Last Initiation" on page 81.)

We are not talking about living in an old body for hundreds of years; we are talking about learning to rejuvenate the body and reverse the aging process. Your body does have the ability to produce new cells. (You have already seen this in yourself many times; for example, when you repair a cut.) Your body is a constantly flowing stream of life. It has a built-in regeneration battery. If you use your mind correctly, you are in charge of how you flow your stream of life.

Of course if you are tempted by the idea that you are not one with God—and therefore cannot determine the consequences of your own actions—and are not in charge of your own body, it is all over. Once you invalidate your divinity in this manner and think you are a sinner, you will give in to helplessness and think, "I cannot heal myself" or "I am weak" or "God is going to destroy me since I am so bad."

Spiritual masters do not think like that at all. They constantly remember who they are. That is the difference. Some of them can rapidly youth or age their bodies at will, and some can even transform them into male or female, a child or an elderly person at will. Babaji is an example of such a master. (Read *Autobiography of a Yogi* by Paramahansa Yogananda.) It should be our purpose for all of us to become spiritual masters.

God is not only love, but God is also *life,* life without beginning or end. God is not the author of anything that is not Himself. In the Book of Ezekiel, we are told that He wills *not* the death of any, but that all should turn to Him and *live.*

The body is the temple of the living God. But remember this: It is possible to weaken the soul's hold on the body with the thought that death is inevitable or with the thought that disease is stronger than the power of God. *Don't ever allow yourself to think that any disease is stronger than the power of God!* This is a departure from Divine Mind.

The Bible presents death as the last enemy to be destroyed. Revelation 21:4 says, "And God shall wipe away all tears and there shall be no more death."

Affirmations

> *I am alive now, therefore my life urges are stronger than my death urges. As long as I continue strengthening my life urges and weakening my death urges, I will go on living in health and youthfulness.*

> *Life is eternal and I am life. My mind, as the thinking quality of life itself, is eternal. My physical body is also eternal. Therefore, my living flesh has a natural tendency to live forever in perfect health and youthfulness.*

> *My physical body is a safe and pleasurable place for me to be. The entire universe exists for the purpose of supporting my physical body and for providing a pleasurable place for me to express myself.*

> *All the cells of my body are daily bathed in the perfection of my divine being.*

> *The more I am good to myself, the more I enrich my own aliveness.*

The Last Initiation

(This section was given to me in India, and I regret I cannot give you the author. It was merely handed to me as is.)

Finally, the concept of immortality implies a harmonization of the entire personality and a transformation of the physical organism as an effective channel of expression of higher values. This may be called material immortality.

There are some mystics and spiritual seekers who strengthen and purify their bodies just enough to be able to experience the thrilling touch of the Divine. They use the body as a ladder—climbing toward a pure spiritual level. On attaining that level, the body is felt as a burden, as a prison house, as a string of chains that holds one in bondage. Dissociation from this "last burden" of the body is considered a *sine qua non* for total liberation. Continued association with the body is believed to be the result of the residual trace of ignorance.

*The above view is based on a subtle misconception
about the purpose of life and the significance of the
body.*

The body is not only a ladder that leads to the realm of immortality of the soul, but it is also an excellent instrument for expressing the glory of Physical Immortality in life and society. It is capable
of being thoroughly penetrated by the light of the Spirit. It is capable of being transformed into what has been called the "Diamond
Body." As a result of such transformation, the body does not appear
anymore to be a burden on the liberated self. It shines as the Spirit
made flesh. It functions as a very effective instrument for creative
action and realization of high values in the world. It is purged of all
inner tension and conflict. It is liberated from the anxiety of
repressed wishes. It is also liberated from the dangerous grip of the
death impulse born of self-repression. Mystics who look on the
body as a burden suffer from the anxiety of self-repression and the
allurement of the death wish.

Material immortality means decisive victory over both these
demons. It conquers the latent death instinct in man and fortifies
the will to live as long as is necessary as a channel of expression of
the Divine. It also liquidates all forms of self-suppression and self-
torture and self-mutilation. As a result, the total being of an individual becomes strong and steady, whole and healthy. There is a
free flow of psychic energy. It is increasingly channeled into ways of
meaningful self-expression. Under the guidance of the indwelling
light of the Eternal, it produces increasing manifestations of the
Spirit in matter.

Happiness Equals Health

Many people think or say, "I won't be happy until I am healthy." This is understandable; yet the truth is that you will be healthy when you are happy. If you read Dr. Deepak Chopra's books, especially *Quantum Healing*, this becomes very clear; he even explains it scientifically. He also makes it clear that unhappiness is due to loss of contact with the source, which means that people forget that they are one with God.

Mother Teresa said that most people are spiritually deprived and that this is the whole problem with the world. This is very important; yet when people are told to become spiritual to be happy, they often rebel. They are likely to think that means they must go back to something such as the church or some kind of dogma. They usually do not want to do so, because they have rarely seen it work for their parents and/or they have been disappointed in religion themselves. This is a tragedy.

Becoming more spiritual is really finding the deeper *self* that is *real*—that part that possesses absolute wisdom and self-knowledge. Dr. Chopra says that in India, finding the "knower" is considered life's greatest adventure. That is exactly why I love to go to India each year! I cherish having the opportunity to be with the great saints who are bursting with joy. In one's spiritual life, this is called the "principle of right association"—placing oneself with the highest beings possible so that one is forced to adapt *upward!*

This past year when I went to visit the great saint Shastriji, Babaji's High Priest, he said this to me as I approached him and his family: "I want you to have intense joy!" That made such a deep impression on me. Did you know that the mother of our great American comedian Robin Williams told him when he was a child

that the purpose of life was to have intense joy? Imagine the blessing of having a parent telling you that at such an early age! Parents,
take note!

> Happiness *derives from the verb "to happen." Happiness
> is to be found simply from observing what happens. If
> you cannot be happy at the prospect of lunch, you are
> not likely to find happiness anywhere. What happens is
> happiness.*
> —Johnson, Robert. *Transformation: Understanding
> the Three Levels of Masculine Consciousness.*

The idea, of course, is to be happy no matter what goes on
around you *and* to know how to be happy without your happiness
depending on material things. You must also remember that all
misery is self-inflicted and that blaming the world for unhappy situations will never work. All this has to do with handling your mind.
Your mind-body system must be connected with pure consciousness. (In transcendental meditation, it is called the "unified field,"
which is the source of all energy fields and fundamental particles.)
When we are then aware of our connection to that, as Dr. Chopra
says, all existence is experienced once again as bliss.

"Bliss," Maharishi, the founder of transcendental meditation,
says, "is ultimately the most powerful agent of physiology."
Maharishi says that any attempt to treat disease or any form of suffering on the physical level is too superficial. Bliss *is* the fundamental nature of the self. The method that Maharishi and Deepak
Chopra recommend for experiencing the state of bliss is to settle
the mind through transcendental meditation.

In my book *Pure Joy*, I list many other methods of spiritual
purification that help you return to that state of bliss. All this does
not mean that you should not try to arrange your life so you are
happy about your surroundings, your job, your relationships, and
your situations. Of course all that is important, but not nearly as
important as the state of your mind. You may be in a job and/or a
relationship that is not right for you, which is definitely not a good
idea. I know many people who stay in dead or destructive relationships because they are afraid to leave. Staying in a relationship you
do not want to be in just because you are afraid to leave is *not* a

good reason to be there. And is it even ethical? Staying in a job that makes you unhappy does not make any sense either. If you do not like the way things are in your life, change them! You may have to leave your job, your marriage, your area, or whatever.

Warning: It may be just your attitude, however, and even if you change all these external things but do not change your attitude, the same thing could come up elsewhere. First try loving where you are, whom you are with, and what you are doing, and see what happens.

Many people are unhappy because they have no idea why they are here or the purpose of their life. Nothing really "hangs together" for them. I could say a lot on this subject, but let's get clear on one thing: the purpose of life is not just to get married, have children, and then die. The purpose of life is to recognize the Supreme, according to my teacher Shastriji. (That is entirely another ball of wax.) This means, of course, that you really need to think about your priorities. Are you, for example, on the spiritual path of becoming all that you can be?

The formula for happiness from my guru Babaji is this: *love, truth, simplicity, and service to mankind.* (He also recommended the mantra "Om Namaha Shivai" for purity.) Do you understand that all work is worship and that you should dedicate it to God daily? This changes everything, by the way. Think about these things.

Readiness and willingness to do any work at any time in any circumstance is the hallmark of spirituality. Spiritual people do it with love and sincerity, without expecting anything. That is why there is always a charm and beauty in whatever spiritual people do. They love to do the work, because the work itself gives them infinite happiness. When we keep worrying about the result, the work loses its beauty.

> *To derive the full benefit of any action, whatever it may be, love for that particular action is absolutely necessary.*
> —Mata Amritanandamayi, *Awaken Children* (p. 260)

This is all great, you might say, but you feel really, really depressed . . . so you cannot relate to any of this. What about that? Depression can be understood like any other symptom and treated spiritually. You need to find the cause of the depression, and for that, you can actually use the same Truth Process in this book.

A Course in Miracles goes so far as to say that all depression (like sickness) is an *idol* that is made up as a substitute for God!

We have found in breathwork that the main cause of depression is the unconscious death urge. As I mentioned earlier, this is a "consciousness factor" that includes your programming on death, the thought that death is inevitable, your secret wish to die because you hate your life, past-life memories of dying, the thought "I am separate from God," and other antilife thoughts. All of that can surely make a person depressed!

My very first client as a breathworker was a real test for me. She came to me very depressed, saying she wanted to kill herself. She was very suicidal and she told me she did not want me to try to talk her out of that. She went on and on and on about why she wanted to die. I listened, but then I realized, of course, that the part of her that wanted to live had come to me for breathwork. If she had truly wanted to die, she would never have come at all. So I focused on that part of her mind. I honored her wish not to push her to live. I just asked her to lie down, breathe, and to simply postpone her suicide for five days, until her next breathwork. I checked on her every day. I did this each session until suddenly, after about eight sessions, she wanted to live. She had breathed out enough death urge in the sessions that she felt different. She later became a dancer. Imagine! Now she is also happily married.

Even if you have what has been called a "fatal illness" and you have a "bad prognosis," let me repeat what Leonard Orr said: "As long as you have one breath left, there is still a chance." And he also reminded us that Jesus took it even further and brought people back *after* they died. For more information on these kinds of cases, read *The Romeo Error* by Lyall Watson. So never give up!

You might say, "Right, okay, I have now decided that I do not want to let a boring job, boring life, or boring relationship ruin my body . . . but how can I guarantee I can get out of these dreary messes?"

Well, what about the *boring mind* aspect that goes before these results? Here is a very interesting statement, again by Leonard Orr:

> *Most people fear eternal life more than they do physical
> death; but what they really fear is not eternal life of*

*their bodies, but the eternal life of their boring minds!
The essential characteristic of a boring person is the
morbidity of the deathist mentality.*

*Conquering death is the basic intelligence test of
spiritual enlightenment.*

Remember: Deathist mentality is unhealthy for human beings.

Influence of Relationships

A relationship can heal you or damage you more, depending on how you play the game of relationships.

You may want your mate to agree with you on everything and back you up no matter what. Or as a mate, you may think that is what you are required to do—agree with him or her and back them up no matter what. This might look like a healed relationship, but what if it is just collusion and codependency that you are creating? If so, watch out later. In other words, what if your mate agrees with you just to make you happy, and what if you are into your ego or "case" at the time? He or she would be supporting your case, supporting your ego, supporting that which will eventually make you sick and destroy you! Now that someone agrees with your case, how will that help you and heal you? It won't! You merely reinforce what you are supposed to be getting rid of. If you reinforce your case with the help of your mate, this will make it *more stuck* and you have the likelihood of getting *more sick.*

The same is true vice versa—colluding with your mate could make her or him sicker. In the book *Love without Conditions,* my friend Paul Ferrini calls this "the Tyranny of Agreement." In other words, the ego cannot conceive that there is any love when two people disagree. If you support behavior that could be hurtful to your mate, this is the ultimate codependency. Peace does not come through the agreement of two egos. The truly healthy relationship has room for disagreement. You can even disagree without upsets. If you listen carefully to a mate who disagrees, you can learn what you need to change to stay healthy.

Married couples often tend to think they must back their spouses no matter what. But what if your spouse is out of integrity?

Well, if you support that kind of thing, you are not only colluding, you are also adding to your own karma!

So where is the balance? How do you support a mate without supporting his or her ego? And how can you handle this without making your mate feel she or he is wrong and that you are being too critical? Ah, very good questions! I have tried to address this in my recent book *Essays on Creating Sacred Relationships: The Next Step to a New Paradigm*. It has to do with knowing what is real and what is the ego. Then, handling that well, it has to do with attitude, grace, enlightenment, and excellent communication skills. Now we are talking about the dynamics of a relationship. Now we are talking about the real *art* of creating a relationship with good dynamics. If you truly love your mate, do not support his or her case, or make it real, or allow him or her to get by with it. Instead, provide the safety net, the love, tenderness, and kindness for this person to feel safe enough to look at what he or she is doing to him- or herself.

You are the mirror, and you offer your mate a new turn that would be healthier than the one she or he is taking. But you must first ever-so-gently help the person see that the way he or she is going may hurt him or her or others. If you point that out in a harsh way, your mate will, however, feel hurt by you and will resist.

When, however, you face the fact that you are the one you live with, you will see it is also you out there you are talking to. (Why do *you* have this situation in *your* vibration?) The mate you are upset with is *your* mirror. What your mate is doing is probably something that was done in your childhood that you need to forgive. Ultimately, working on your own case is the answer; and being willing to get help with that is a good idea. Tell your mate that you actually want him or her to point out to you where you were wrong. Who wants a "yes man" anyway? (Only someone who is totally insecure.) How boring!!

Try this attitude: Welcome criticism. Be glad when someone points out your faults. They are healing you. This is surely a big opportunity for you to grow. Welcome feedback. It is good for you. If people fabricate things about you, insult you, or inappropriately abuse you, you should be unshakable even then and not let it ruffle you. But of course, you should look to see how you attracted *that* and try to keep from attracting that result ever again. My guru

Babaji said to us, "Be not concerned with praise or abuse. Do your work!" This advice has helped me so many times as a leader.

I have known many married couples whom I also knew pretty well as single people before they met each other. Before they met, they were each strong in their own right, with tremendous potential, often making great contributions. However, after moving in with each other, they more or less "caved in" on each other and became dependent and weak. Often they sold out, giving up dreams and not becoming at all what they could have been. I have often seen them almost destroy each other. Why? I have written several trainings on relationships that answer this question.

Obviously, the point is that a relationship should strengthen you—not weaken you. You should be happier because of the relationship, not more miserable. You should *expand* because of the relationship, not contract. You should get financially more prosperous as a result, not less. You should get healthier, not sicker. This is the goal, the ideal. However, to handle everything that comes up in a relationship and to keep growing stronger, enlightenment is required. Instead of saying it feels impossible, try reading *A Course in Miracles* and see why the above is not happening for you.

If your mate does happen to become ill, the way you handle that also affects the outcome. If you go into agreement with the illness, make it real, and give it undue attention, you are both reinforcing it. If you start feeling very sorry for your mate and worry and treat her or him like an invalid, you only make it worse. That does not mean you must be cold and ignore someone who needs support. The support he or she needs may not be what you thought, however.

Encouragement and love without making someone more helpless is a good start!

It is best to see the person as healed. Keep imagining her or him without the condition and help the person heal by using the techniques in this book. Your confidence in a miraculous outcome can make a difference that is huge. I *know* it is hard when you are in love with someone and you are panicked, thinking he or she might abandon you by dying or something. Perhaps you will need help yourself to hold the highest thought.

One of the main ways you can support someone who has become ill is to make sure the person does not forget to do the Truth Process just as soon as the symptoms surface. Do not wait until your mate gets a full-blown illness with a major "diagnosis." Also study the *CIM* pamphlets that explain how Jesus healed people. Try to align with his mind. Where would I be today if people had gone into agreement with my arthritis? I would not be writing this book, probably.

I know many people that stay in destructive or dead relationships because they are too afraid to leave. Staying in a relationship because you are too afraid to leave is not a good reason to stay. And is it even ethical? If you are lying to yourself and being unethical by staying, your chances for getting sick are greater.

People often ask me if they should leave a relationship immediately or wait and see if it ever clears up. This is not for me to decide. What I do tell them is to pray for this relationship to be healed *or* for something better for both of them. Then, either way it is a win. I tell them to pray for *Divine Right Action*. Of course, there are many cases in which conditions suddenly shift and miracles happen. We all know of cases in which people stayed too long and totally regretted it. I know that one must pray a lot on these points.

Just the other day I received a letter from a woman who wrote, "It is strange how I have been hanging on to this extremely painful relationship; and now I feel so *relieved* that it is over. I am like a new person." (As for me, I know if I had stayed in my first marriage, I would likely be sick right now and there would have been none of the trainings I wrote and led.)

Miracles can happen even in the worst scenarios. This takes two persons' total commitment. And the only way to have a perfect relationship is for both people to be willing to experience their own perfection. So I would say that commitment to self-improvement and spiritual enlightenment must be the top priority for both for the healing of the relationship to happen. Denying and pretending will only be destructive to the body.

Some relationships have been destroyed because the couple never learned good communication habits. There is a vast area for improvement in this area for all of us. It is worth spending the time to study effective communication. I know I could have stayed in some relationships longer if I had known how to communicate better.

Influence of Communication

What you do *not* say could make you sick or keep you in pain. Werner Erhard, the founder of EST, used to say to us, "What you cannot communicate runs you." I was always a very talkative person, and after I heard that, I talked even more! However, I wondered whether it was *true* communication. Was I really saying my truest feelings? I began saying them more. I began really telling people what I wanted and what I thought. That seemed to work. Then I began writing. This form of expression helped me even more. I thought, "Oh, boy! I am really expressing myself well." I thought I was on top of it. But I was not really.

The next level was facing what I was in denial about and admitting that. That was scarier. It was shocking to me to find out that there were things I was afraid to say. It all came to a head on a trip to Australia during which I had some trouble with my hip. A guide told me I was starting to process genetic ancestral material. Then she shocked me by proceeding to tell me that my grandparents from Sweden, long-ago dead, had appeared to her. They wanted me to know a big secret existed in my family, and she even told me what it was. I was stunned, but I knew it was true because right away it kind of explained a whole section of our family life that I had never been able to understand. She told me it would take several months to process that family pattern.

Well, I wanted to speed things up, so I had some cranial-osteo work in Spain by Geraldine. She intuitively worked on my gums for one whole hour. Then she told me some anger would come out and I would no longer be able to withhold anything; I would get out of denial about many things I needed to communicate. But I *still* did not think I had anything to communicate that was so big. I was really unable to see it. But within the next few days, it all came out. I knew suddenly with whom I had to communicate and about what I had to communicate. But it was still scary. I thought there would be anger. I was so afraid of anger that to keep peace, I was with-holding a lot of stuff. So I was faced with how to communicate this delicate material that truly affected my business. Very tricky. First I had to write copious faxes about my fear of communicating. Then I spent days being "very diplomatic." One day I was not so diplo-matic. It was rocky, but I hung in there. After all this, I felt much, much better physically. My energy in my body went way up. My power and happiness dramatically increased. But I should have done it long before it had become so hard to make changes. I waited far too long. My business was "sick" by then.

Maybe you are sick or in pain because you are too afraid to say to your mate, "Today I really feel like leaving this relationship." There is a great chance that if you just say it and you feel heard, your desire to leave will also change.

I have heard of a number of cases in which people finally began communicating something to a person in the family—when that person was on her or his deathbed! I guess the feeling was "Well, since he is going to die anyway, this cannot kill him." I know of a guy who finally told his mother as she lay dying about something she had done his whole life that really bothered him. She was so sorry he had not told her sooner because the whole thing was a complete misunderstanding, a communication problem. She had meant just the opposite of the way he took it. The incident had negatively affected his whole life for nearly forty years. Problems start from poor communication, but you need good communication to clear up the problems.

For years in our community, we tried the way of *direct feedback*. This was an overcompensation for withholding. This was better than "stuffing it," but I kept noticing that people still got on the defensive unless the feedback was worded perfectly. The person receiving the feedback often felt attacked, and instead of really hearing the communication, began to find a way to attack back with similarly strong feedback. We plowed through this and we got bet-ter at it—better at giving it and better at receiving it. I prided myself at being able to "take criticism." I felt I had enough self-esteem. But

I never felt satisfied with the whole thing because for many, it was too devastating.

I also noticed that for the really delicate, hard, sensitive things that people were still afraid to say, they would tell someone else rather than the "offending" person directly. This would get back to the person for whom it was really intended. That person would confront the one who had said it to someone else. The person who had said it would deny it, back down, or say, "Oh, I did not mean it that way at all. So-and-so misunderstood." This drove me nuts. I tried to give a lecture on all this to the community at a summer event. But I saw little change that year.

Then I read an article about a group in San Diego studying communication. A man had developed what he called "compassionate communication." He recommended that a person first say, "What I feel is . . ." and then "What I want is . . ." For example, instead of saying, "You don't handle this issue about the children. You never deal with it at all. You avoid everything. I don't think you are a good father and you don't support me!" you would say, "What I feel is sad because I cannot get this issue about the children resolved. What I want is resolution by tomorrow night. So I need for you to think about it and tell me your desired result by then."

It is really important to hear out everyone in a family and relationship. Give them space to say everything without interruption. Then say "Thank you" instead of being on the defensive. This discharges the energy, and they will be able to drop the upset. You will be surprised at how much better you will feel physically after these simple procedures.

Another good thing to remember is that when a person is upset and coming at you, it is best to just listen and see if you can find one thing with which you agree. You might not agree with most of it, but start out by saying, "I can see your point about . . ." or "I agree with . . ." and then stop to integrate this alignment.

Try reading the book *You Just Don't Understand* by Deborah Tannen to learn more about the difference in male and female communication. I have also written more about this in the book *Essays on Creating Sacred Relationships*.

PART IV

Methods of Spiritual Healing

Spiritual Healing Techniques

The following is a method of healing I have developed over years and years of study. It is so simple that now I wonder why it took me so long to get it. Perhaps it was because it has taken me a long time to unravel my addiction to Western medicine, and that had to go out first. Then I had to integrate all my years of breathwork, training in India, and what *A Course in Miracles* says. After that, I kind of "reduced it all down" like a sauce.

There are three main parts to this self-healing technique:

1. Finding the cause of the condition (the *real* cause, the metaphysical cause)

2. Confession of the addiction (the addiction to those negative thoughts causing the condition)

3. Spiritual purification methods (for releasing the thoughts that cause the condition)

1. *Finding the cause:* This is accomplished through what I call the Ultimate Truth Process, which you can do in writing. In this way, you become your own Sherlock Holmes, telling the absolute truth to yourself on paper. You must let go of the thought "I don't know," because that blocks your ability to access the information. You *do* know the cause of your condition. It is in your mind. You must just let the responses come up to consciousness. A writing process helps you do that. On paper, write the following:

A. *The negative thoughts I have that are causing this condition are:*

B. *My "payoffs" for having this condition are:*

C. *My fears of giving up this condition are:*

D. *My most negative thought about my body is:*

E. *My most negative thought about myself is:*

F. *When this condition first began was:*

G. *What was going on in my life at that time was:*

See page 99 for an example of this Truth Process. This technique is called self-analysis.

2. **Confession:** Recognizing the above data is an addiction (something I stubbornly hang onto), I confess to God and another person that I indulge regularly in the above ego thoughts and I have been refusing to let go of them. (Read to another person the above list you wrote, and standing before your altar, read it to the Holy Spirit.)

3. **Spiritual purification methods:** Some examples include the following:

Affirmations	*Indian sweat lodges*
Prayer	*Writing*
Breathwork	*Silence/seclusion*
Chanting	*Visiting an ashram*
Meditation	*Head shaving*
Fasting	

See my book *Pure Joy* for the other methods and all explanations.

It is good to have a buddy who also understands these techniques to do a reality check with you. The ideal reality check person would be your personal breathworker.

Another process you can do with your breathworker or buddy is a verbal Truth Process such as a "sentence completion technique": "I will allow myself to be healed when . . ." Keep repeating this phrase and fill in the blank. I am not talking about a time span here. You are confessing to your buddy what you think needs to happen before you are safe enough to let go of this condition.

For example, "I will allow myself to be healed of _____ (when I am sure my mother is okay first)," or "I will allow myself to be healed of _____ (when I feel I have suffered enough over my sister's death)," or "I will allow myself to be healed of _____ (when I experience my perfection)."

A skilled breathworker would then take you deeper and have you say, "I will know my mother is okay when . . ." or "I will feel I have suffered enough when . . ." or "I will experience my perfection when . . ."

These "answers" will give the breathworker necessary information about why you won't allow yourself to be healed *now*. Sometimes you may be setting up impossible situations for yourself, such as "I cannot let myself be healed because my mother is not healed." Perhaps your mother (or brother or other family member) does not want to be healed and you will therefore have to wait forever. Waiting for family members to go first is a mistake. You go first and set an example. The breathworker will help you process and breathe out unrealistic expectations.

The following is an example of the Ultimate Truth Process (writing):

Condition—Extremely Dry Skin

1. *The negative thoughts I have that are causing this condition are:*
   - I don't drink enough water.
   - A part of me is "dead."
   - I want to be like my grandmother.
   - I don't want to be too seductive.
   - I don't want to be touched too much.
   - The exact negative thought causing this condition is that I can be more like a man and be like my father.

2. *My payoffs for having this condition are:*
   - I don't have to be too feminine.
   - I can keep men away.
   - I don't have to be too sensual.
   - My biggest payoff for having this condition is that I don't have to be seductive.

3. *My fears of giving up this condition are:*
   - With beautiful skin, I would seduce men more and have to be a real woman. (My father wants a boy, not a girl.)
   - I would have more sex and more touching, and I would be distracted by that.
   - I would attract too many people if I were totally radiant.
   - My biggest fear of giving up this condition is that I would be glowing and saintlike. I am afraid of perfection.

4. *My most negative thought about my body is that it won't do what I want.*

5. *My most negative thought about myself is that I am not perfect.*

6. *This condition first began when I was a teenager.*

7. *What was going on in my life at that time was my father had died.*

I want to say a few more words to explain the meaning of *payoff*. A *payoff* is something that one gets out of a condition that is neurotic or something negative that one is trying to "prove."

If the payoff is too great, the person may not want to give up the condition. Furthermore, to give up the condition, the person must also be willing to give up the payoffs. Therefore, it is important not only to understand what the payoffs are, but it is even more important to learn that one does not need these neurotic payoffs. Below I list some more examples of payoffs. Note that the word *symptom* is interchangeable with *disease*.

- *Attention*
- *Punishing oneself with the condition because of guilt*
- *Keeping people away*
- *Using the symptom to prove that one is helpless, bad, worthless, unable, not perfect, not good enough, a failure, and so on*
- *Punishing a mate or parent to try to make them feel he or she is not good enough or is bad*
- *Using the symptoms as a way of holding oneself back because of fear of moving forward*
- *Using the symptom as a form of conflict because one is addicted to conflict*
- *Using the symptom as a way of trying to prove that there is no God*
- *Using the symptom as an excuse to be angry*
- *Using the symptom as an excuse not to work*
- *Using the symptom or disease as a cover-up or distraction to avoid what is really going on*
- *Using the symptom as a way of sabotaging one's life, career, or relationship*
- *Using the symptom as a way of deadening oneself because of fear of feeling and/or fear of life*

You can handle these issues in healthier, less neurotic ways. For example, you don't have to be sick to get attention. You can learn that self-punishment in the form of sickness is not necessary. You could forgive yourself instead. You could change jobs and find something you love to do rather than getting sick to get out of a job you hate, and so on. You can actually leave a relationship instead of getting sick to get out of it.

Some examples of *fears* people might have about giving up the disease or symptom including the following:

- *Fear that if one should give it up, one might have to be responsible*
- *Fear that if one should give it up, one might have to succeed*
- *Fear that if one should give it up, one might have to face something*
- *Fear that if one should give it up, one might have to move forward and be powerful*
- *Fear that if one should give it up, one could no longer get even*
- *Fear that if one should give it up, one would have no more excuses*
- *Fear that if one should give it up, one might have to be happy*
- *Fear that if one should give it up, one might end up with a relationship and then one would have to handle love*
- *Fear that if one should give it up, one might end up alone*

You may think you do not have any fear of giving up the condition, but if you still have the condition, you still have the fear. When you work out the fear, you will be ready to give up the condition. (See the section on the fear of healing under *A Course in Miracles* section.) So the first step is to identify the fear and the next step is to give up the fear. Change the thoughts that cause the fear, and breathe out the feeling of fear.

Prayers for Healing

I am quite willing to share with you the prayers I use for healing, but I feel that you should ultimately work out your own prayers so they have more personal meaning to you. It took me a number of years to get this right for myself. For one thing, for me to get back into prayer, I had to work out my case with religion and all my disappointment around religious theology. After leaving the church, rebelling, and reentering spirituality through breathwork, I had to find my way again.

When I met my guru Babaji, he allowed me to write to him all my prayers in the form of letters. I decided that one purpose of a guru is to permit you to bare your soul to him. So that is what I did. I shared with him all my problems, laid them at his feet, and asked for guidance. Usually I had an emotional release during this process and my energy would shift. Then I would experience a change in my body. I actually did this for years, but now when I think of it, these prayers seem kind of crude and embarrassing to me. But in a sense, it was the best I could do and was my way of giving it to the Holy Spirit. Later, after Babaji entered his final Samadhi (conscious departure), I continued to write him and still do to this day. I place the prayers on my altar until I feel the issue clears. It *still* works for me. But it works better now because I have learned to compose the prayers in a more responsible way.

1. *I state my gratitude and forgiveness.*

2. *I state my problem.*

3. *I try to confess how I created this problem myself—what ego thoughts, negative thoughts of mine were in operation.*

4. *I lay those at his feet.*

5. *I ask for the ability to see the problem differently.*

6. *I choose new thinking to counteract my old thoughts.*

7. *I ask to have the new positive thinking fortified.*

In this way, I take more responsibility for my case and show the Divine that I am willing to do something about it. I am not saying, *"Oh, please do it for me."* Begging for something is a lower form of prayer. Gratitude is the highest form of prayer.

Sometimes I add other steps. I sit before my altar and speak aloud to Babaji, Jesus, the Divine Mother, and so on, all of whom represent the Holy Spirit's mind to me. At first I felt silly doing this and really embarrassed. But the results were fantastic, so I went ahead anyway. The desire to communicate with the Masters is essential to opening the door to their presence. It must start with you. You must *invite in* the Holy Spirit.

I learned a five-part prayer as a child in the Lutheran church that is really excellent:

1. *Opening*

2. *Forgiveness*

3. *Gratitude*

4. *Petition*

5. *Closing*

1. **Opening:** In this part, you "set the stage" and get into the proper frame of mind. I do this by repeating mantras or by reading from *A Course in Miracles* workbook the lesson for today. You could also read from the Bible or from any spiritual metaphysical book that is important to you.

2. **Forgiveness:** In this step, you state the following:

A. What you want to be forgiven for.

B. Whom you want to be forgiven by.

C. Whom you want to forgive, and so on.

3. **Gratitude:** Now you state, with deep feeling, everything for which you are grateful and everybody to whom you are grateful, with love and appreciation.

4. *Petition:* At this point, you actually ask for guidance and help with specific problems. (Here I would read specific prayers for the healing of the body. See the example below.)

5. *Closing:* Finally, you again read the scriptures. Text from *A Course in Miracles* is ideal.

Example of Number 4: Petition

You would read the following at your altar:

Regarding my condition of gastritis (for example):

> *I take responsibility for creating this condition caused by negative thoughts of mine, such as . . .*
>
> *I lay this at your feet. I allow you, the Holy Spirit, to undo all my wrong thinking that caused this condition and those thoughts that keep me from giving it up.*
> (Read the negative thoughts from your Truth Process as a confession.)
>
> *I now choose to think that I can create* peace *instead of this. I place it all in your hands. I ask you to help release me from this and raise it from me.*
>
> *I ask to be taught the right perception of the body.*
>
> *I pray for release from the* fear *of the miracle healing. I pray for help in the cause of that* fear, *which is my addiction to the thought of separation from God.*
>
> *I do not want to keep this error.*
>
> *I now ask* (the part of the body affected; in this case, intestines) *to cooperate and let go. I cooperate with you and follow you* (the mind of Jesus). *I believe that you know what to do and will guide me. I choose union with you. I am willing to receive the solution.*
>
> *I have total willingness to have God's will for me, which is perfect happiness and perfect health. I know that in you, in your mercy and will, that I will be saved from this.*

I therefore completely release the thought that this
cannot be healed. The completed results of Jesus Christ
now manifest for me in this situation. This is the time
for divine completion!

If the above prayer does not produce results, try this one. Begin by placing your palms down as a symbolic indication of your willingness and desire to turn over any concerns you may have to God. The following are some examples:

Lord, I give you my anger at . . . (palms down)

Lord, I would like to receive your divine love for . . .
(palms up)

Lord, I release my fear of never being healed of . . .
(palms down)

Lord, I receive now your certainty that I can be
healed of . . . (palms up)

Lord, I surrender my anxiety about my . . .
(palms down)

Lord, I receive now your peace about my . . . (palms up)

When you do these palms-down and palms-up movements, spend some minutes in complete silence and wait until you feel something. Do not rush this process. Allow God to commune with your spirit.

Note: Prayer *does* have the power to heal. Scientific studies actually prove it. Dr. Larry Dossey, cochairman of the National Institutes of Health, has reported many studies in which patients have responded remarkably to prayer. In fact, prayed-for patients were five times less likely to develop complications or need antibiotics. So if you are very ill, not only should you try the prayers above, but why not get yourself on a prayer list and let people pray for you? It works.

Breathwork and Healing

Breathwork, or conscious breathing, is a physical, mental, and spiritual experience. The physical part consists of connecting your inhale and exhale in a relaxed rhythm (with no holding at the top or bottom). The spiritual dimension of conscious breathing is the heart of the matter. One purpose of breathwork is not only the movement of air but also the movement of *energy*. The dynamic energy flows that are experienced during breathwork are the merging of spirit and matter. The energy flows are the process of filling your body with pure life-energy and cleaning your mind and body of tension and impurities. You can also remember and release your birth trauma in breathwork, which makes a huge difference in your life. It should always be conducted by a well-trained breathworker. (See the appendix for information on locating one in your area.) Only after one has become a breathworker and has passed certain levels of expertise should one try to breathwork oneself.

This kind of conscious breathing gives you a great self-healing power! We think of breathwork as the ultimate healing experience, because your breath, together with the quality of your thoughts, can rapidly heal you. We have seen symptoms, from migraine headaches to ulcers to sore ankles, disappear completely as a result of breathwork. Respiratory illnesses, stomach and back pains have disappeared. Frigidity, hemorrhoids, insomnia, diabetes, epilepsy, cancer, arthritis, and all kinds of other manifestations have been eliminated. Many of these conditions seem to have been caused or prolonged by birth trauma. Leonard Orr said, "People get stuck in birth trauma symptoms and then develop medical belief systems about them." He added, "Doctors can then become mother substitutes to support infancy patterns."

In breathwork, we see people go through physiological changes in ten minutes that other people stay stuck in for years and from which they may even die.

On the other hand, breathwork creates a safe environment in your mind and body in which symptoms from the past, such as childhood illnesses and patterns, can act themselves out. It is a good idea to keep in mind that these symptoms are temporary and relatively easy to eliminate with uninhibited breathing. (Some people have created diaper rash, for example.) But if, in your mind, you are afraid of childhood symptoms or resent them, you may inhibit your natural healing powers.

If you have a lot of fear, it is a good idea to consult physicians you really trust, as well as spiritual and mental healers, until you work out the fear of self-healing. They will help you get out of the traps in your mind.

Breathwork is not for people who retreat from life in fear or who desire to curl up and die—unless they want to retreat from that pattern! Breathwork is for people who desire to live fully, freely, and healthfully in spirit, mind, and body. We do not claim that any cure is permanent, because human beings have the power to re-create the symptoms. But *Permanent Healing is* the goal and *is* available. However, it is up to the individual to accept the opportunity.

Breathwork creates a safe environment in the mind and body that enables clients to become free of all negativity; however, processing negativity can be overwhelming at times. That is why we recommend you take it gently, starting out with only one session a week. We also recommend that you make the whole process of spiritual growth easier by participating in a spiritual community that assists you effectively and supports you in whatever changes you may go through. Cultivating the philosophy of Physical Immortality also gives you optimism and makes conquering all difficulties an adventure instead of a bewildering tragedy.

I could have presented many examples of healing by breathwork. Obviously, it would require many volumes to relate the complexities of all the personal case histories of people we have helped. But even if you labored through them, they still might not help you. There is really no substitute for trusting your own intuition about your body and a community of friends who can add their wisdom to your personal healing.

The purpose of breathwork actually was not for healing in the beginning, but healing turned out to be a valuable by-product. The purpose of breathwork is to acquaint people with a dimension of spiritual energy that they may not have heretofore experienced. When people experience this process, they can connect their illness or pain with the original negative thought out of which it was created and thereby take total responsibility for causing it. Some people are therefore completely able to let go of the condition instantaneously during the session. It literally gets pumped out of the body with the breath. Others may gradually let go of it during the following weeks after the session. The breath is the cleanser of the body, as the yogis have always known.

It is usually possible to come out of breathwork in a perpetual state of health and bliss, but the path might be rocky. For example, when people experience their actual birth in breathwork, they may begin reexperiencing various stages of infancy and some feelings of helplessness. In my own breathwork, I noticed that I never went through something I could not handle; the harder things came up only when I was strong enough to take them. But these rocky periods did not bother me because the more I worked out my birth trauma, the more energy I experienced. This kept increasing and still is. For the rocky parts, I was able to remember that "this will pass." Also, breathwork ultimately raises your self-esteem; when that happens, all areas of your life are affected positively.

People may avoid breathwork because they experience fear when they even hear the word! It is not that breathwork *adds* to your fear, however. One of the purposes of breathwork is to *release* fear. Feeling fear when you think of breathwork just shows you how much fear you have suppressed in your body since birth. Breathing it out will be a great relief. I personally would never commit my life to something that was dangerous. I have learned that it is more dangerous to keep the birth trauma suppressed in yourself. Now it has taken the process to a whole new level that feels even more pleasant and sacred.

The following information is taken from the book *Rebirthing in the New Age,* by Leonard Orr:

> *The birth trauma is your introduction to the world. It is the beginning of the "The Universe is Against me"*

syndrome. There are preverbal thoughts and there is preverbal intelligence. Your thinking began before you were able to verbalize these thoughts—in other words, before you were born. Therefore, when you were born, you were able to make sophisticated conclusions about that traumatic event. The womb is a comfortable place where all physiological needs are supplied. When we are pulled from this ideal environment, we experience a considerable amount of pain and discomfort. Probably 90 percent of our fear originated with the birth trauma. Some of the generalizations we might have made at birth are:

"Being outside the womb is unpleasant."
"I cannot trust people."
"If this is what life is like, I don't want to be here."
"People are out to get me."
"I can't get enough air (love), nourishment, etc."

The birth trauma is one of the reasons most people don't like to get up in the morning. The bed simulates the womb experience. In the process of awakening, the memory of birth pains are stimulated to near-consciousness. These near-memories trigger the fear that you will have to reexperience being born again. Warm baths and showers also stimulate womb experiences. (Some people choose even a hospital as a substitute for the womb or heaven.) Even something like smoking can symbolize being back in the womb . . . trying to get to the comfort of having the lungs full as they were in the womb.

Impatience, hostility, and susceptibility to illness and accidents can sometimes be traced back to the birth trauma. Many people feel either too hot or too cold and never experience lasting physical comfort during their entire lifetimes because of unpleasant birth experiences. We view the traditional theological description of heaven as a symbolic description of the womb. What people are really after when they seek "heaven" is to get back to that feeling of the womb. People want to go back to the womb because it has not been very pleasant since they came out; and it is unpleasant because of the negative decisions they made at birth, which produce negative results. The breathwork experience was created to enable you to go back and dissolve all that.

Other Alternatives

Emotional Release

I have usually found that when I need to let go of any stubborn pattern or symptom, I must let myself break down and cry at some point to get the physical release.

Of course, this is easier to do during breathwork. Having a breathworker present to keep you breathing through it helps the energy move. If I do not have a fellow breathworker, I can usually get myself to cry by "wet breathwork" on myself in the bathtub. However, I do *not* recommend that you try it on your own until you have reached a certain point in the breathwork process and your breathworker, having trained you, feels you are ready. I point it out, however, as it is something to work toward and look forward to.

There are other ways to get oneself to cry and have an emotional release. I can also make myself "crack" by throwing myself facedown on the floor in front of my altar and repenting my mistakes. Another way I do it is by lying down on the bed and talking aloud to Jesus until I finally let go and cry.

Since I am a writer, the fastest thing for me to do is to write to my guru Babaji and confess my case on paper. You do not have to be a professional writer to write a confession to God. Usually when I get to the bottom line, I start to cry. This cleansing always works for me.

Another thing you can do is sit across from a friend and say, "Something I feel sad about is . . ." and "Another thing I feel sad about is . . ." If you are getting down to the bottom line and telling the real truth, usually the sadness will finally manifest in tears and you will feel better. You can often heal yourself of symptoms by having very deep crying sessions (especially symptoms of cold and sinuses).

The point is that not only does one have to change one's thoughts to be healed, but it is also of particular importance to breathe out the negative mental mass. Feeling the feeling is also part of this process. Feeling fear and sadness rather than stuffing them is one of the secrets of staying healthy. I may be crying because I am sad about a situation, but I also cry often as a way of repenting my mistakes. It is humbling to feel the sadness of one's errors. It helps me to admit aloud to God that I have been wrong in my thinking (which is obvious or I would not have the symptom). If you do not feel well, you have chosen wrongly.

To some people, it might seem easier just to go to the doctor and get some pills. But believe me, pills are only temporary relief. If you don't get the consciousness factor that causes your symptoms, the symptoms can easily return, possibly in a worse form. *A Course in Miracles* says that pills are forms of a "spell." They work if you *believe* they work, but putting a "spell" on yourself like that does not work in the long run. Ultimately, you do not need pills if you surrender to the healing power of God. However, on certain occasions, if you have too much fear of spiritual healing, you should not judge yourself if you take a medical treatment. But the goal should be to wean yourself eventually of that. Feeling your emotions and releasing them is one of the keys.

Movement

Sometimes it helps to say prayers and mantras with movement, especially if you can walk on the beach or on a relatively quiet path. It is very good to play a tape of mantras (with earphones) and walk very fast while repeating them. This really moves the energy in your body and cracks your case. I find it much more interesting and effective than gymnastic workouts.

If you ever feel too sick or out-of-it to walk fast, move, or even chant, at least put the earphones on your head with the mantras playing as loudly as you can stand and prostrate yourself in front of the altar, even if you must crawl to get there. That is a symbolic "movement" of humility.

I hope that you will call your breathworker before you get too sick. By the way, if you have symptoms, don't cancel your breathwork appointment! That is the exact time you need to go. *Get moving* toward your breathworker.

Another form of movement that is not too overwhelming when you have symptoms is the following: Put on some music of African drums. Just stand in place and shake your body. Close your eyes and don't worry about how you look. Keep doing this and then lie down and breathe with your breathworker. Your breathing mechanism will be more open and productive as a result of that simple movement.

If you find exercise too strenuous and inappropriate because you feel too awful, maybe you should follow your intuition and not force yourself. Perhaps something as simple as the above will get you started. Later you can try something else nice such as sacred dance or an activity that has meaning for you.

Recently, I experimented with Watsu therapy, movement done underwater. I have found this to be *very* effective. I strongly recommend it as a healing technique. Watsu therapy is a healing art, and because of the water, the body can easily assume positions that would be very difficult to assume outside the water. The spinal fluid is stimulated in such a way that the natural healing powers of the body are enhanced. The therapy requires minimal effort because the Watsu therapist is in charge of moving your body. So you could really feel helpless and still get the benefit of the movements. After the session, you will most likely feel like moving again by yourself. It is a nice transition. Often when you feel sick, the last thing you want to do is move, even though it might help. In this case, the resistance is handled because the Watsu therapist knows how to move you, and the positions are not hard to assume under the water.

For more information, contact Two Bunch Palms Resort in Palm Springs, California, or Harbin Hot Springs, California.

Diet, Health, and Healing

There are so many opinions on this subject that you could easily read a hundred different books and get a hundred different opinions. You can feel crazy after a while, trying to figure it all out. For me, the subject of health and nutrition was one of the hardest things in my life that I had to work out for myself. That was because *(a)* I was born on the kitchen table, *(b)* I was born in the food belt of the world, and *(c)* my mother was a home economics teacher so I had to learn innumerable "rules" about food that were supposed to make me healthy.

In the end, I rebelled against it all because I felt I was going mad. I had to write the book *The Only Diet There Is* to heal myself so I could relax even enough to eat at all. I had been so obsessed with this subject for so many years that I had tried too many different "diets," too many different ways of eating, too many food plans, too many nutrition programs, too many nutrition products—*too* many even to think straight.

And in the end, I reduced it down to the fact that I *liked* being a vegetarian. It feels right to me physically, morally, and energetically. I also like the results. And yet, that is just another opinion: *mine!* You must find out what works for you. I have been a vegetarian for over two decades, and it makes me happy. But now that is getting hard to do. Since this book was finished I moved toward being a fruitarian. This is really working for me!

I honestly feel the whole subject is best summed up by fellow Immortalist, JoAnna Cherry. She expresses my sincerest feelings even better than I can. The following paragraph is from the chapter she wrote called "Divine Self" in the book *New Cells, New Bodies,*

New Life by Virginia Essene and others. I recommend this book, obviously.

> *Are you eating what feels most right for you at this*
> *time? Foods are all thought forms, just like our body;*
> *and we do have the ability to transform any food—with*
> *our thought, love, light, intention—to a frequency that is*
> *totally beneficial to our body. But until we fully*
> *empower ourselves with this ability, our body will love*
> *some food more than others. Raw and organic fruits*
> *and vegetables, soaked nuts and sprouted seeds and*
> *beans hold the greatest natural light. Many wonderful*
> *new substances are available today also that can*
> *enliven and lift your body. Try and just listen to your*
> *Spirit and the highest desire for your body, and follow*
> *that.*

I discuss this topic more fully in the book *The Only Diet There Is,* which teaches you how to keep the weight you want by the power of your mind, and also in my book on Physical Immortality, *How to Be Chic, Fabulous, and Live Forever.* In that book, I discuss some of the research on which diets are believed to enhance longevity.

On the subject of vegetarianism, again, certain Immortal teachers say that if you eat meat, you participate in the karma of killing, which does not cooperate with your desire to be Immortal. But the *other* argument is that is just another thought that you can change! So you see, you must just think for yourself. You do have to determine whether or not your thoughts are powerful enough to overcome these aspects; you must decide how you feel morally, and so on.

You might need to consider this: if your thoughts are clear enough, you can drink even poison and not die. But would you test this out? Kahuna masters have done so. I met one. But most of us don't go around testing this. We don't go around proving we can drink poison. Well, then, are we ready and able to process poisonous food? Why make it hard for yourself? Also, which foods do you think are poisonous? Maybe everyone should actually read *Diet for a New America.* When you read that and find out what *really goes on* when meat and poultry are processed, you might not feel like eating any of it again. You should investigate all this yourself and decide for yourself. I would not recommend that you rely on what you were taught in school on this subject! How do you know that was the highest thought? It probably was not. Nor do I want to insist that my opinion is the right one.

I do have to admit, however, that I have been influenced somewhat by great minds who wrote about these subjects. Here are some examples:

Jesus: And the flesh of slain beasts in his body will become his own tomb. For I tell you truly, he who kills, kills himself; and who so eats flesh of slain beasts eats the body of death.

Buddha: Let the Bodhisattva who is disciplining himself to attain compassion refrain from eating flesh. Meat is food for ferocious feasts: improper to eat. . . . so said the Buddha. If, bereft of compassion and wisdom, you eat meat, you have turned your back on liberation.

Leonardo da Vinci: Truly, man is the king of beasts, for his brutality exceeds theirs. We live by the death of others. We are burial places. The time will come when men such as I will look upon the murder of animals as they now look upon the murder of men.

Percy Bysshe Shelley: It is only by softening and disguising dead flesh by culinary preparation that it is rendered susceptible of mastication or digestion, and that the sight of its bloods, juices and red horror does not excite intolerable loathing and disgust. Let the advocate of animal food force himself to a decisive experiment of its fitness and, as Plutarch recommends, tear a living lamb with his teeth and, plunging his head into its vitals, slake his thirst with steaming blood. When fresh from the deed of horror, let him revert to the irresistible instincts of nature that would rise in judgment against it and say, "Nature forced me for such work as this." Then, and then only, would he be consistent.

Henry Thoreau: I have no doubt that it is part of the destiny of the human race, in its gradual development, to leave off the eating of animals as surely as the savage tribes have left off eating each other when they came into contact with the more civilized.

Leo Tolstoy: Vegetarianism serves as a criterion by which we know that the pursuit of moral perfection on the path of man is genuine and sincere. It is dreadful that man suppresses in himself, unnecessarily, the highest spiritual capacity . . . that of sympathy and pity towards living creatures like himself . . . and by violating his own feelings becomes cruel. And how deeply seated in the human heart is the injunction not to take life.

Annie Besant: People who eat meat are responsible for all the pain that grows out of meat eating, and which is necessitated by the use of sentient animals as food . . . not only the horrors of the slaughterhouse, but all the preliminary horrors of railway or ship traffic, all the starvation and the thirst and prolonged misery of fear which these unhappy creatures have to pass through for the gratification of the appetite of men. All pain acts as a record against humanity and slackens and retards the whole of human growth.

I was quite glad that I was a vegetarian myself before I found this book. I do admit that this book influenced me to stay with it. Notice if what they said makes you angry. If you are still a meat eater, it might make you angry. These great minds would probably propose that your anger is a result of eating meat! Please do not invalidate my whole book just because you might be angry at these quotes. I did not say that you *must* give up meat. I am merely saying that it is a good idea to think it over and be really clear on your decision. You might realize that you have been brainwashed by school, parents, television, and nutritionists. Maybe you have never considered your own spiritual feelings. Maybe you have never tried to be a vegetarian, and maybe you would like it. Who knows? As for me, I prayed about it. I said, "If this is right, take the desire for meat from me. I am willing for Divine Right Action." I left Bali and did not want red meat or poultry after that. Now when people spend some time with me they say they automatically start eating less and less and they are glad.

I have been discussing food from a standpoint of health maintenance. It is also true that certain diets can help the healing process—but that is true only *if* a person truly wants to get better and is not sabotaging her- or himself. My experience is that abstinence from food (fasting) has the most beneficial effect on producing healing. In my opinion, fasting is a very spiritual matter, and when done properly, a profound healing and a "spiritual gift" usually occurs at the end. You must process your mind when you fast; the mind is, after all, what makes you sick. Food is often used to suppress the very part of the mind at which you should be looking. When you are not eating, you cannot go on suppressing what you need to see because what you need to see will just confront you. A good book on fasting called *Are You Confused?* explains all different types of fasts. You do not get hungry on the master cleanser, for example—and it works. Many other books on fasting are available at your local health food stores.

In general, you could say that eating less is very good for you. You have much more energy to help keep you healthy. It has already been proven that you live longer if you eat lightly. It is a good idea to start cutting down and to cut down more every year. But do it gradually. Some people, however, feel a real loss if you tell them not to eat so much. They actually feel a loss of love—probably because their mother showed them love by giving them food. It might also remind them of the sadness of being taken off the breast. For some people, food is like a friend, and they use it as a substitute for having real friends. The same is true for cigarettes. But once you get through these notions and get into another reality—the reality of eating lightly by choice—I think you will really like it.

Many people are just eating the same way their parents ate. They do not think of whether or not that is what they really want to eat. I notice that when I eat a very light meal and enjoy that, many people cannot stand it. They urge me to eat more. They worry about me. They try really hard to get me to eat more, more of what they eat. They cannot shut up about it. They get stuck in medical belief systems that convince them that I am not going to be okay. Or maybe they don't want to face the fact that they would like to be able to eat less. (Or at times, maybe I had them set up as my "mother.") Nevertheless, you need to experiment. Chances are, a new world will open up to you when you start thinking for yourself on this subject. Source your *own* rules!

If you are dealing with a severe health problem and you feel that you need support from a healing diet and a strong healer, you might consider the program of my friend Michelangelo in Milan. (I acknowledged him earlier for helping me heal my gastritis after my sister's death.) His healing program uses the highest vibration *vegan* foods along with very strong reflexology. This regime, although fanatical to some, has proven extremely effective for

many. People with near-fatal diseases have been cured at his center.
You can reach him at his institute: phone 0039 02 89 50 2085; or
fax 0039 02 895 15555.

Clearing Karma That Causes Disease

In the book *Star Signs* by Linda Goodman, there is an important
true story. A friend of hers was really shaken when he was told he
had contracted a rare disease for which there was no cure. The disease, he was told, would gradually paralyze him over a year's time.
What this amazing man did was to accept responsibility for his
karma. He realized that in a former life, he had caused someone, or
several people, to be paralyzed. The reaction of his original action
was an attempt to balance the scales under karmic law, which is
quite impersonal. He might have caused such a karmic debt by
being a hit-and-run driver, running from the scene of an accident
and leaving the victim paralyzed, and so on, or by deliberately injur-
ing someone in a sport such as boxing or whatever. He might have
been one of those in Rome who threw people to the lions.

Upon facing his karmic debt, he meditated on polarity action
and made a decision. He resigned from his high-paying job and
offered his service for a very modest salary to a crippled children's
hospital in a nearby city. He read aloud to children, assisted them
in physical therapy, and even performed unpleasant janitorial tasks.
He started to forget about his own illness. Three months after he
took that work, he noticed that his pain was substantially less.
Later, when he returned to his hometown for a routine check, the
doctors were amazed to find that all signs of the fatal disease had
disappeared. It was a *spontaneous remission*—the medical term for
a miracle.

Another example might be that of a barren woman who lifts her
karma. If a woman wants a child and is told that she cannot conceive or bear a child for whatever medical reason, there is often a
karmic cause for her dilemma. She may have abused children in a
former life. She may have been an illegal abortionist who damaged
women. So in this life, she adopts a child. A physician friend of the
author told her that statistics as high as 75 percent to 85 percent
show that of women diagnosed as barren discover they are preg-

nant *after adopting*. When a woman learns the karmic lesson of Atonement by taking in a motherless child to give it love, the karmic burden is lifted.

Goodman, Linda. "Déjà Vu." In *Star Signs*. 120–121.

Perhaps you need to do some very deep thinking about this; ask yourself if you need to apply this to yourself in any way.

Once I took a young man to India to see my gurus. This young man had serious intestinal problems, and in fact, ended up with a colostomy at a very young age. He consulted my gurus about his karma. My gurus were reluctant to tell him because they did not feel he would handle the facts well. He pushed them and pushed them to tell him. Finally, one said he had been a drug pusher in a past life and had been responsible for the destruction of the bodies of some of the people to whom he had sold drugs. Later he asked me what to do. I told him to work with teens to prevent them from using drugs. He did not like the assignment and got angry, just as my teacher had said he would. In his case, he was not ready to face the truth in himself. Apparently, he needed more time to integrate this information.

Recently, one of my wealthier, sophisticated acquaintances from the "old days" of breathwork was having an exceptionally difficult time recovering from her sister's death. She got sick herself and suffered terrible dizzy spells (which I did not know about because I had lost track of her). Where had she gone? To an ashram! I saw her afterward, and she was healed. She said it was the best thing she had ever done in her life. Initially, I was surprised she had gone alone, because she is very sophisticated; I did not think she would put up with ashram life. But then I remembered that she had gone to India with me years before, so she did have the power of ashrams built into her consciousness. She had taken our seminars in the old days and she had had breathwork. And so, her higher self remembered what was good for her. She did not complain to me once about the facilities. All she kept saying was that it was the best thing she had done for herself.

I have written much about the benefits of ceremonies and experiences in ashrams. For more information, please read *Pure Joy*. One of my great teachers, Shastriji the High Priest, blessed me with the privilege of publishing some of his speeches in that book. In those speeches, he carefully explains how and why chanting heals you, how and why head shaving is so powerful, and why the ceremonies work.

Nobody is saying that you *must* shave your head at an ashram. Nobody is saying that you *must go* to an ashram either. These are merely choices that are available if you want results more quickly. The question is, "How long do you want to suffer?"

Usually people do have resistance to going to an ashram. They say they don't have time or they could not stand the conditions, and so on. That is understandable, *but* what are your priorities? Do you want to end up in a hospital? Once you are in an ashram, it is actually very adventurous and fun.

I don't want to give the impression that you go to ashrams only if you are sick. Nothing could be further from the truth. Ashrams are places of worship. The more you go, the better. This is also the way to stay in bliss, to stay healthy. It is also the best preventive medicine I know. People so often ask me where I get all my energy, and so on. Quite often when students go with me to India and experience the ashrams where I had my training, they say, "I finally understand where you are coming from!"

Just being around the great souls who live in those ashrams is exhilarating. They transmit spiritual energy to you all the time. Also, Babaji has trained certain yogis to do a healing technique called *jara*. You lie down and the yogi sits near you with a bundle of peacock feathers tied together. He strokes your body with those while repeating secret mantras taught to him by the guru. (The yogi can do this only if the guru says he is ready and the yogi has prepared himself through a long, special process of purification.) This treatment is very effective. I was recently given the right to use jara on people for healing.

All kinds of healing treatments are available in the world. Don't limit yourself. You will find the right one when you are ready to let go. But always remember that it is very important to do the other steps first—the Truth Process and confession.

Seeking Spiritual Counseling

If you are stuck on something, it is often good to talk to someone who is more intuitive than you are at the time. You should always trust your own intuition, of course. But when you are sick, you may not trust your own intuition because you feel "out of it"; or you might feel that your intuition is almost shut down. That is temporary, of course, but when you are sick, your ego *is* roaring; when your ego is roaring, that is hardly the best time for intuition. However, you do have to use your intuition enough to know to whom you need to talk. At least you need to know someone you can fully trust who has tried that healer, that clairvoyant, or that spiritual guide.

I became a great believer in trying many forms of healing because I thought, "Why limit myself?" I have had no guilt or qualms about consulting others when I have been stuck, especially when a past life was affecting me and I could not see it or process it by myself. Sometimes I easily figured out what to do or had a revealing dream. But often I grew impatient. Sometimes I just needed to hear what a person who was clearer than I at the moment could see. One told me that I had a karmic break from a past life in Atlantis, where I had allowed myself to be experimented on with lasers for the upliftment of humanity. Apparently, we overdid those experiments. This information helped me and I modified my healing methods accordingly.

Other times I have had intense "cranial shifts" that were not really headaches per se, but they were painful. I knew they were important, but I had a difficult time. I was told by a spiritual guide that I was having exceptionally intricate work done on my electromagnetic fields, and as a leader, I must be willing to accept the ordeal. Had I not discussed this with a colleague, I may have gone into a panic. I might have felt I needed to run out and get an X ray or something. Or worse, I might have imagined I was getting a brain tumor like my sister had. By having this support and feedback, I relaxed and I learned to know my body better. I learned to recognize the symptoms that indicated that kind of spiritual change and how they were different from other symptoms.

Of course, I must reemphasize that you can get the answers yourself if you need to. In some situations no spiritual guides are around. Once I did get quite scared. I thought I was getting a brain tumor like my sister. I had terrible headaches, and I became paranoid because such headaches were highly unusual for me. I prayed a lot. During the night, I dreamed the following dream: My skull was cut off by someone and set aside so that I could look into my brain. I knew I was seeing my own brain, and that was rather eerie . . . but I needed to see it. There was absolutely no tumor there, but there was a place where there was "drainage," and a piece of gauze was over that. In my dream, I shouted, "What is *that?*" The answer came as this: "That is the negative thought you have had that 'something is wrong with you.' That negative thought is draining out." I was pretty calm during the dream, but later I found it shocking that I had seen my own brain. Then I became grateful. I knew it was a gift.

The Ashram as a Place to Be Healed

Since you are reading this book, I assume you are committed to self-healing and you are willing to do anything to stay out of hospitals, if possible! Let's hope you never create anything really serious; on the other hand, this can happen to the best of us, especially during very stressful times.

If you really want to expedite the process of healing, especially if you think it is not working or is going too slowly—I would suggest you get yourself to an ashram. If you are not up to going to India, there are also many in the West. I list them in the appendix for you. You can also call this number for information: (719) 256-4108.

An ashram is a place set aside especially for purification. It is usually in a location that is rather remote and "out in the elements," where you can receive more spiritual power. The central focus is a temple in which you pray, meditate, and chant many hours a day. The important thing about an ashram is this: not only do you have the energy available, thanks to the guru's grace and location, but you also have a totally different routine that is so different that it makes your ego collapse. Often this is just what you need to break up the pattern of sickness. Staying home, going through the same old routine day in and day out, is often too "soft" and in many cases will not move the ego out. But when you are forced to participate in a routine that is totally different, in a setting that is totally different, you change, you are released—especially if the spiritual energy is strong enough. The rituals and ceremonies at an ashram help cleanse and purify your mind and body.

The subtle ego is very hard to conquer, especially by only your own effort. A guru can transform your mind into a powerhouse of inexhaustible energy. You feel safe enough and strong enough to win the battle of your ego in an ashram. For example, I have seen people who were stuck with a lot of anger, which was destroying their bodies. But they were afraid to give up the anger because they had it wired up that they *needed* anger to survive. (So they thought they would die if they gave up their anger.) Of course, this is irrational and the opposite is true, but the ego tricked them. In daily life, they were too scared to drop their anger. And yet, at an ashram they felt so safe that they became like lambs . . . the sweetest things imaginable. There, for the first time in their lives, they felt safe to give up anger.

I have seen people heal themselves of major life-threatening illnesses in an ashram. The constant spiritual energy pushed them through it. I have said the following repeatedly, and I still stick with this statement: If I had a serious illness, I would immediately go to an ashram and shave my head. I have done this even for illnesses that some people would not call serious—but for me, they were conditions that were hard to heal. So rather than struggling and struggling with my ego, I merely shaved my head. This definitely brought everything to a "head"!

Interesting Notes on Healing

Sickness always has an element of escapism in it.
                    —Chopra, Deepak. *Unconditional Life.*, 9.

Complete healing depends on the ability to stop struggling.
                    —Chopra, Deepak *Unconditional Life.*, 24.

Spiritual connection is the hidden variable in health.
    —Ferguson, Marilyn. "The Paradigm of Proven Potentials."
                                    New Sense Bulletin.

In almost all such cases involving cancer, spiritual and psychic growth is being denied or the individual feels that he or she can no longer grow properly in personal, psychic terms. This situation then activates body mechanisms that result in the overgrowth of certain cells. The individual forces an artificial situation in which growth itself becomes physically disastrous. This is because a blockage has occurred. The individual wants to grow in terms of personhood, but is afraid of doing so. Often the person feels like a martyr (to his or her sex, for example) and is "unable to escape."
            —Roberts, Jane. *The Nature of the Psyche: Its Human
                        Expression.* A Seth Book. 71.

In cancer, a normal working cell decides that it no longer wants to function in contribution to the whole.

*Instead of being part of the support system, the cell goes
off and builds its own kingdom. That's a malignancy.*
—Williamson, Marianne. *Return to Love.*

The point being made is that this is merely a reflection of our
making an ego, a separate self, a false self to replace God.

The following are two examples from the great book *New Cells,
New Bodies, New Life* by Virginia Essene:

*In brief, you are in a Holy Coordinate Point. Let me
assure that these incoming energies bring healing to your
soul and physical genetic body patterns. For this healing
to happen, the cells must receive and retain more Light
and be released of many past restrictions, limitations,
and imperfections caused by the present life. The paired
chromosomes must be cleansed at least four generations
back. (pp. 2–3)*

*Health is an area in which everyone needs to claim
responsibility for themselves. You DO have power over
your body. From infancy you were told that you have no
power over your body. You were told that you must
always check with someone else about health and well-
being. You have the innate ability to take charge of your
body. You DO replicate your body daily. You create the
same body because you expect to see the same body. If
you wish to change it, simply intend that when you
wake up there is something new to greet you. (p. 178)*

(On rejuvenation—mental level) On the mental level, bringing
forth Immortality means releasing all the ingrained limiting beliefs
about your body and replacing them with unlimited truth.

*(On affirmation) I now give up death. I give up all aging
of the body, all illness and any other effect that limited
thought has had upon my physical form. I give up the
idea of being any age. I am ageless and eternal. I give up
funerals and funeral parlors and grave sites. I give up
the idea of leaving life. I joyously accept eternal
aliveness now.*

(p. 68; in the chapter titled "Divine Self" by JoAnna Cherry)

I hope to inspire you to read that whole book. The last chapter has a lot to say about healing; that is, intradimensional healing, sound healing, and quadrant healing. It requires personal study and is well worth it.

> *Illness is some form of inner searching. Health is Inner Peace.* (p. 15, A *Course in Miracles*)

The following are some quotations from Marianne Williamson's lectures and book, *Return to Love*, which I recommend strongly:

> *Disease is loveless thinking materialized.*

> *Health is the result of the relinquishing of all attempts to use the body lovelessly.* (A healthy perception of our bodies is one in which we surrender them to the Holy Spirit and ask that they be used as an instrument through which love is expressed in the world.)

> *Sickness is not a sign of God's judgment on us, but our judgment on ourselves.* (If we think God created our sickness, how can we turn to him for healing?)

> *Forgiveness is the ultimate preventive medicine, as well as the greatest healer.*

> *Illness is a sign of separation from God. Healing is a sign we have returned to God.*

> *By shifting our awareness from body identification to Spirit identification, this heals the body as well as the mind.*

> *There is a healing force within each of us, a kind of divine physician. This force is the intelligence that drives the immune system. The Atonement releases the mind to its full creative power.*

The following is another quote from "'No' Law of Healing" by Catherine Ponder in the book *Dynamic Laws of Healing:*

> *Denial is the first law of healing. Through denial you withdraw from your mind the negative beliefs and emotions that have played havoc with your health. If you can put a thing out of your mind, you can put it out*

of your body. Since denial dissolves, eliminates, erases
and frees, it is your "NO" power of healing.

Any prayer or statement that helps you say, "No. I do not accept this appearance as necessary or lasting in my life," is a denial. (In her opinion, to mentally affirm a healthy condition without first denying and destroying the negative emotions that caused your ill health is like attempting to build a new house on a site already occupied by an old building. Say no to an incurable diagnosis.)

Say, "I refuse to accept this diagnosis." (She suggests that you do not believe anything anyone tells you about your health unless they say you are going to get better!) Read chapter 2 of that book for further information.

In the book, Catherine talks about a friend of hers who was told that her daughter, who had speaking and hearing problems, was "intellectually disabled." When the child was four years old, her diagnosis was "developmentally delayed." Fortunately, the girl was not in the room when this diagnosis was given. The mother was told that the child should go to a special school. The mother told the daughter she was not going to acknowledge this. In fact, she did not tell the father, friends, or relatives. She sent the child to a normal school, and the girl did all right. At age eight, the child had to have an operation. The mother was told that the girl would never be able to have children. The mother again did not accept this and told no one. Later the girl grew up as a wonderful, normal person and had two healthy, normal children.

So the point is, you can use denial to help others!

My Summary on Healing

To Those of You Who Really Want to Know When You Will Be Healed

You will be healed when you are ready to be healed. You will be ready to be healed when you believe you deserve it. You will believe you deserve it when you are ready to stop punishing yourself. You will stop punishing yourself when you give up guilt. You will give up guilt when you believe you are innocent. You will see you are innocent when you remember who you are. You will remember who you are when you stop making up the ego. You will stop making up the ego when you want bliss and peace more than anything else. You will want bliss and peace when you are sick of being sick . . . and when you see what a waste of time it is to be in hell. The choice is yours. (One teacher said you must want liberation as much as a drowning person wants air.)

Permanent Healing is merely going back to who and what you really are. It is easy and natural; the only reason it *seems* hard is because you must let go of addictions—addictions to thoughts that cause the conditions. It seems hard to give up addictions because you think they control you and that you are not in control of them. In my opinion, an addiction is a stubborn refusal to give up something. It might be merely a stubborn refusal to give up a thought causing your condition. When you face your stubbornness and refusal as being something you choose, you know you can choose otherwise.

A Course in Miracles tells you that you must say, "I see no more value in this." That means you must also admit that you get some kind of payoff from your pain or illness. You receive some kind of neurotic value out of this condition, and now you are willing to give up that payoff. For example, maybe you must decide you don't need this symptom anymore as a way to get attention. You no longer need this symptom as a way to punish yourself. You have enjoyed enough attention and you feel punished enough! Perhaps you have learned you can get attention in a healthier way. Or perhaps you feel you have balanced your karma and you can go on to something else.

But what if you could forgive yourself *sooner*? Then you would not have to go to the trouble of punishing yourself for so long. To forgive yourself sooner requires a basic understanding of who you are: You are *love* and your sins are not real. You must know that you are not a bad person. You are actually magnificent. You are a child of God. You are divine. You are not a sinner. Your disasters are not sins; they are mistakes. A mistake merely means "missing the mark." A mistake is a slip when you temporarily forget who you are. God does not make your errors real, because God knows you were just having a nightmare. Nightmares are not real. The ego is a nightmare. But since the ego is not real, the error is not real. Therefore, you do not deserve to be punished and you do not need to create illnesses as a form of punishment. If God does not make your mistakes real, why should you? You do not make your child's nightmares real. Do you want your children to make their nightmares real? Of course not.

Innocence is the Answer.

Since I am innocent, I do not need to suffer.

Since I am innocent, I deserve to be healed.

Since I am innocent, I can let go of all the pain and disease.

Since I am innocent, the Holy Spirit in me knows the solution.

Since I am innocent, it is safe, right, and holy to have a body.

Since I am innocent, I can be really happy.

Since I am innocent, I can give myself love and keep it.

Since I am innocent, I can have all that I need and want.

Since I am innocent, I can handle a lot of energy.

Since I am innocent, I can trust myself to do the right thing.

Since I am innocent, I can be defenseless.

Since I am innocent, I am at peace.

Since I am innocent, my body responds to really feeling good.

Since I am innocent, I can totally relax

Since I am innocent, I can become wiser and wiser.

Since I am innocent, I can say no without losing people's love.

Since I am innocent, I can enjoy food, money, and sex.

Since I am innocent, I can enjoy everything.

Since I am innocent, it is okay to have things.

Since I am innocent, I have nothing to worry about.

Since I am innocent, I can leave situations that are not good.

Since I am innocent, fun is natural.

Since I am innocent, life is natural.

Since I am innocent, success is natural.

Since I am innocent, I do not have to age and die and
punish myself.

Since I am innocent, I can live as long as I choose.

Since I am innocent, I can be in the kingdom of heaven here
and now.

Since I am innocent, I can be close to the spiritual masters.

Since I am innocent, I can make a big contribution to humanity.

Final World
(For Now)

If you read hundreds of books on healing, the common denomina-tor will surely be *love*. That is obviously the secret of all successful healing.

The healer must love the patient; and the more loving the healer is, the faster the patient will heal. But the patient must return to self-love and love for God and life. That is the key. If you are the patient *or* the healer, meditate on love.

When I was working in Japan the first time, I heard an incredible true story. I was told of a man who developed cancer of the lungs. What he did on hearing that diagnosis was amazing. Every day he sat before his altar and expressed *appreciation* for his lungs, for life, and for God. He constantly meditated on appreciation. By doing this, he experienced a complete miracle healing. The healer who told me this story explained to me that *appreciation* is one of the very highest vibrations for healing.

If *appreciation* is the ultimate vibration for healing, imagine how it could also be preventive medicine. Perhaps if we sincerely appre-ciate people and things and life, then perhaps we would not even get sick. Perhaps if we appreciated and loved ourselves all the time, we would not have the problems we have.

Think about it!

Health in the Future

The famous trendsetter and marketer Faith Popcorn has been called the Nostradamus of marketing. In her book *The Popcorn Report*, she discusses how we all thought, worked, and lived in the 1990s. She states that self health care is the future. We will become our own experts. We will counterpoint the advice of a homeopathist, a reflexologist, and so on.

Faith Popcorn predicts the following:

> *Medical knowledge and alternatives will cross cultures in a way we have never seen before. Homeopathy, Refloxology, Acupressure and Acupuncture, Biofeedback and Holistic Medicine will move from the fringes to the mainstream of medicine. Even newer-sounding approaches such as Aromatherapy, Herbology and Ancient Indian Ayurvedic Medicine will be incorporated into traditional treatments or stand on their own as preferred courses of action. (p. 67)*

Of course, it is obvious to me that breathwork will be included in that list! She also feels that entertainment and travel will be health- and longevity-obsessed:

> *Beyond health spas will be "Mood Spas," Universal Energy Gyms, Mind and Spirit Reunions, including therapeutic cruises that slowly take you to healthy places, in an effort to heal your body, touch your soul, and bring you back, twice blessed. (p. 68)*

She says we may not yet be ready to admit aloud that our goal is truly to live forever . . . but we will pay anything to stay alive. Well,

I did admit out loud that I wanted to live forever when I wrote the book called How to Be Chic, Fabulous, and Live Forever. I was really daring and ahead of my time as usual. I was happy to see that she calls "Staying Alive" trend number seven.

Interesting Tidbids from The Enquirer

According to University of Michigan researcher Lois M. Verbrugge, the five most common health problems for middle-aged men are:

1. High blood pressure
2. Arthritis
3. Hearing impairment
4. Chronic sinusitis
5. Heart disease

The five most common health problems for middle-aged women are:

1. Arthritis
2. High blood pressure
3. Chronic sinusitis
4. Hearing impairment
5. Hay fever

According to Louise Hay, who wrote *Heal Your Body*, the metaphysical causes of these conditions are the following:

- High blood pressure: long-standing emotional problem not resolved
- Arthritis: feeling unloved, criticism, resentment
- Hearing impairment: not wanting to hear something
- Chronic sinusitis: irritation, especially to someone very close
- Heart disease: lack of joy, hardening of the center of love

Doesn't that mean, therefore, that we are a society of need in the area of love, that we are stuck in resentment and criticism and we don't want to hear? Are we so addicted to favoring money and position that we forget the most important things in life? Are we so rigid that arthritis is popular? Are we so unaware that we need to resolve emotional problems that we have to shoot up our blood pressure to get our own attention? All symptoms are to get your attention and to wake you up. The trouble with the symptoms mentioned here is that by the time you create *these*, they could be really hard to reverse. Prevention is the whole point. Wouldn't it be better to take the time to handle emotional problems before they turn into a diagnosis like these?

The whole point of Louise Hay's book *Heal Your Body* is that you must first work to dissolve your mental cause. Her book explains the common mental causes of conditions. Carry this little book with you and pay attention. Don't become one of the statistics mentioned in *The Enquirer*. The problem with reading these statistics is that if you go into agreement with them, you can easily create them in your body. What you believe to be true, you create. So you must decide that this will not become true for you; and of course, you must carry through with the spiritual purification procedure to prevent it.

PART V

My Most Difficult Initiations as a Healer

Going toward the Stargate

Sometimes the challenge of being a committed lightworker is shocking, even to me. For example, I never dreamed I would have to go through a kind of "crucifixion" in France. Actually, it was a spiritual "opening" or initiation, but it felt like a crucifixion. Oh, yes, I did ask for liberation in this life—and Immortality—so I should not be surprised, I guess. Also, I have an assignment in this life to be a pioneer on the "front lines," so I should not be surprised. But it would be a lie to say I was not shocked at what happened.

I started the journey January 1, 1992. I was aware that the big day, January 11, was coming up, and I should have known I would be profoundly affected. This was networked as a special day, like Harmonic Convergence, for an evolutionary leap. Lightworkers gathered around the globe and linked up to welcome the dove, the symbol of Planetary Ascension. Under the direction of Archangel Michael, three stargates were to be opened, one at each pole and one satellite stargate that revolves around the equator. You might think of it as symbolizing the Holy Trinity, as formlessness and spirit. This I already knew from the *World Ascension Network Newsletters* and by word of mouth, through my colleagues in the Consciousness movement. My newsletter stated that "through the newly opened stargates flows a Christic 'super glue' that serves to hold the etheric perfect to the physical imperfect. Over the course of the decade, and in specific order, all blueprints grids and ley lines will be set into place." Fine; I was into it. I agreed to fast on January 9, 10, and 11, and I would definitely meditate at the agreed time, 11:11.

It so happened that around this time I had been instructed by my teacher in Spain to move to France. I was having a really hard time with this assignment, because I don't speak French and I have a

137

huge block to learning it. All my guides did agree that I needed to be in Europe during this time to help support these changes. I had always been good about fulfilling every assignment, so I set out for France to tour and see where I should locate. Fortunately, my teacher Shastriji in India had instructed one of my students, who is trilingual, to accompany me. Another student, who is French, also accompanied us for the first half of the trip. The only directions I received on the phone from a guide was to go to Bordeaux and find a man named Peter. This mystified me. I was not given a hint where to find him, and everyone said I was nuts for going to Bordeaux. I could not tell one town from another. I knew nothing about France, it seemed. I merely told my students that we must go there.

Halfway there we stopped to visit some people we knew. I was shocked to see them living with no central heating—only a fireplace stove. I was *freezing*. This added to my resistance, which then really began building up. I felt helpless, not knowing French, and I did not know where I was going. I did get it in my head, though, that I must find the place the Dalai Lama had visited. I had no idea where that was either, but I knew I had to go. The first night we stayed in a delightful town called Salat. I was so cold that I had to sleep under my fur-lined coat. I could not imagine people living like this in modern times: who needs this? But we did find the Buddhist center, and we did find a man named Peter there, so I felt I was on the right track. But why did my guides send me on this route? The people I met through Peter started showing us a number of castles. They kept wanting me to see these castles from the 1200s. I thought, "Who needs this? I am a futurist." The more castles I saw, the deeper I went into resistance. I felt forced backward in time and I hated it. At that point, I could not imagine living in France. I was told I needed the astral influences, but what kind of bullshit was that? I felt my guides had not given me enough information. Later I realized that had they done so, I would never have taken this trip. Things got harder and harder and harder. Sometimes we would be in a little French town, and we were the only ones in the hotel— always freezing. It seemed that everyone ate goose liver and went to bed very early because there was definitely nothing happening.

I told Alan I had had it, and I wanted to go farther south where it was warmer and that we could stop and visit his mother. Besides, the rental car was getting too expensive and I was getting too resistant.

We headed south and I was so pleased to see a glimpse of pale sun and to meet Alan's mother that I felt happier. I could not speak a word of French to his mother, and therefore was shocked that she told him she had never been so affected by anyone's presence in her life. She did not want me to leave. I was simply amazed by her impression, because I felt I was still totally resisting France. How could she feel so good about me? This kind of woke me up as to who I was again, and I felt rather guilty. Why couldn't I always be loving, no matter where I was? I had been so many places and had so much fun. What *was* my problem with France, anyway? Everything seemed too difficult. I was not used to this at all. I could not understand what was going on. I had lived in Peru in the Peace Corps and had taken breathwork to Russia and Ghana, Africa. So why on earth was I this resistant to France? Finally, I could stand it no longer. I called my teacher.

I confessed it. I told him that if this was a test, I felt I was flunking it. I told him I could not get my mind together and so on. He informed me that I had a past life in the year 1213 in France and I had failed to complete my important mission because a war had broken out. I needed to visit the area of Avignon and St. Remey, where I would get a lot of answers.

Well, I had been incredibly close to the right places. As it turned out, we had to return the car to Avignon. I had a very adverse reaction to that town. The popes had escaped there once. I guess it is a powerful town, but for me, that is where the hell really began. One afternoon I was walking the streets as my teacher had told me to do. I was looking in a shop window, and I suddenly lost my vision. Everything turned black. I was alone and I was sure I was fainting. Suddenly, I grabbed a light pole and squeezed my nipples very hard to stay in my body. I was swaying and I could not remember where my hotel room was. But miraculously, it was right in front of me, so I ran to my room and cried hysterically. I had enough sense to realize my past life was coming up—but I had been through past lives before. Why was this one so much worse? I insisted that we get out of that town the next day. I could not stand it. I sent a fax to Spain and the whole fax arrived totally black . . .

We made it to St. Remey in a borrowed car. The keys got locked in, so I had to stay; I could not escape this time. But I was quite interested in this town. After all, it was the home of Nostradamus.

So I headed to the Nostradamus Café to report the key situation, but it was Sunday. This was complicated. No hotels were open for the winter, of course . . . except an old chateau on the outskirts of town. It was very cold. Alex and I checked in. (Alan had stayed with his mother.) So there we were—the only guests again . . .

That night I had a very unusual dream. It was the beginning of my opening, but I still did not understand what was going on. I dreamed that I saw a serpent, cut up in pieces. Suddenly, a painter came along, got the pieces, and made them into a breathtaking painting. The painting was so lovely that I could not get over it. It seemed to have been painted by one of the impressionists. Well, after all, I was in that area of France.

I knew I was going to have to stay in town two days, but I was in bed the whole time. I spent the two most difficult days of my life in that chateau, which turned out to be on property that had belonged to Nostradamus. At that point, it was January 7 and 8. I was doing conscious breathing like mad, alternating dry and wet. Alex had to take care of me, because my cranium began shifting wildly; the pain seemed absolutely intolerable. My bones were on fire to the point it was too intense to tolerate. I could not let go of the thought "This is too hard!" and I felt I was going crazy. (Vincent van Gogh went crazy in that town and cut off his ear!) Alex gave me body work, and I cried and cried and cried. I thought death would be easier. I told Alex that if my mind were to go too far left, I would be insane, and if it went right, I would die. I was searching for a hairline down the middle. The ordeal began to seem like the drama of Faust and the painful struggle to dethrone the ego. I had been through initiations before, I had been through cranial shifts before, and I had certainly felt my bones on fire before—but *never* like this.

Then I recalled that Ram Dass said that as you get more spiritually connected, more difficult matters come up. I had not wanted to hear that. But now that sentence was helping me stay sane enough to begin to recite to Alex what I could remember from *A Course in Miracles*, which I had forgotten to bring with me for the first time, of course. I was able to access the lines I needed somehow. That seemed to be the only thing that kept me sane. If I had not had that and if I had had to rely on religious dogma right then, I would have become insane like van Gogh, because that is what got him—the sacrifice and suffering aspect of religious dogma, it was said.

Apparently, he went mad trying to cope with that. But *A Course in Miracles* saved me instead. That and, of course, breathwork. Later I was told that my guides and teachers all deliberately pushed me to the limits.

I was able to directly experience how my ego could resist a solution—the ego always does. It is like the devil tempting someone to think no solution exists. This part of my mind made me feel utterly helpless. But I kept on doing breathwork, which saved me. My ego began losing its supremacy, but it forced a huge battle. I finally remembered the part of *CIM* that says that the Holy Spirit is the only true therapist, because the Holy Spirit is conflict free. I started shouting, "The Holy Spirit in me knows the solution." And the solution was to keep inviting the Holy Spiriit to replace my ego.

I remembered that *CIM* said that the ego is insane. I was having an ego attack, but I did not know why until long after the whole experience.

On the third day, I had absolutely enough of that place. I told Alex we must make it to Provence and get me to an acupuncturist. However, I could not even sit up in the car. I started sweating and my clothes became soaking wet. I was out of it, but I dragged myself to this wonderful acupuncturist. When I saw him and began stripping down, I suddenly took my shirt and wrung it out in front of him; the sweat in that one shirt made a huge puddle on the floor. I guess I made a "big splash" in his mind as well, because he took it all very seriously after that. I told him I was not sick but that I was having a spiritual opening. He said he could see that. He told me that my fire energy was on total overload. He worked on me a long time.

After that, I checked into the finest hotel I could find—where Cézanne used to stay. At least it was restored and warm, and best of all, I could get CNN! Being able to see that for the first time in months helped me. I realized I was homesick. But that was nothing compared to the rest of the process.

It was January 9. I began sweating and sweating again. Alex had to change my sheets often, every hour and all during the night. I never got out of bed for two more days. By now, my teacher Jose, who was "monitoring" the whole thing, sent a message from Spain that all was well and that I must go through this. He still did not tell me why. He said the energy I was getting would benefit me and everyone in contact with me. But I felt like killing him . . . literally.

He was pushing me too far. It was still too much. Did he have *any* idea how much this trip was costing me? that I had nearly gone insane? that I had nearly died and had a horrible time? I literally felt I would *never* recover. I was stuck on that thought for a whole day too. I felt wounded, permanently injured. Alex had to take care of me every second because I could not move.

And then finally it was the 11th, the day they "unlocked the gates of heaven." At least I had done well with fasting, because I could not eat a thing for days, had I even wanted to.

At 11:11, I began meditating. The fire had calmed down. I had stopped sweating; but then I began to cry and cry and cry. I felt as though I was being ripped open, something like St. Theresa wrote about: "God has ripped me open." Frankly, it felt more like wild lions to me. I failed to see the rapture of it. I could not stop crying. That night I dreamed a man was killed by a wild lion. The father of the man blamed the siblings for the death. I took the siblings into my room and reminded them that they were not to blame. (I was reminding myself that others were not to blame for this battle I had been through.) In the second part of the dream, I was in the Himalayas. White snow was everywhere. Suddenly, off in the high peaks, I saw a huge red circle "pulsating." It was fresh red blood. I shouted, "What is *that*?" I was told it was a pack of wild lions during mating.

The day after 11:11, I decided to go to Madrid and face my teacher head on. I was still mad at him. Alex had to go back to Barcelona. In the Marseilles airport, I kept chanting, "I will not faint!" In Madrid, I called Jose immediately. Surely he knew I was mad at him, because for the first time ever, he invited me to his home. When I got there, he poured me a brandy to calm me down. He was so loving and humble that I completely forgot I wanted to kill him. He said that I actually did not have to live in France—just go there and clear my past lives. I could have sworn he had told me to *live* there. I know he did. But if he had just said, "Go to France to clear," I would have been like a tourist. I would never have gone that deep.

He told me he had to clear me because I had to be in charge of many healers in the future when great epidemics were expected. Then he told me I was not yet "done" in France; I had to go to Portiers. I told him there was *no way* I was going back there that year. He would never tell me who I had been in that past life or those lives. Maybe it was better. I felt half dead in his presence. But he kept telling me to connect with the good work I had done back then. I kept dreaming of towns in France burning during a war . . .

The last night in Madrid, Adolfo had a dream. He and I were looking at a picture of Babaji. Suddenly, we looked at the sun and that very picture appeared in the sun and became alive. Later we were in the house, and Babaji suddenly came through the window, as a huge flame directly from the sun, and entered my body. I guess I slept through that; however, Adolfo said I was filled with flames from the sun and Babaji was inside me. Then he apparently materialized next to me and began speaking broken Spanish the way Adolfo speaks broken English. (Babaji always told us that if we see him at night in a dream, he was actually there—because we cannot make up dreams about an avatar.)

The next morning Jose called to say good-bye and told me to go where there was sun! He and Babaji were obviously in cahoots over my process! He also read a poem he had written for me, something about letting go of the bitter taste of that experience. So I did. But I had to go back to France the next year.

On that trip, I took two female companions with me. When we arrived at the home of Joan of Arc, we became rather sick and began shaking. During that trip, I was saner and did not have to go to bed so much. However, I definitely needed to see an acupuncturist. I told him I was in town to clear my past lives. He suddenly ran upstairs and got a big fat book on the history of France and started reading to me in French about some king. I thought, "What possessed him to open to that part? Was he channeling? Was I that king?" I cannot remember any of it except that he read to me in French for a half hour while I was under the needles. He was determined that I should know that era of French history. I did not understand what he was saying, but my translator summarized it. At the time, I knew it was perfect. Right now I cannot remember any of it.

After all that, I went to India. At the end of my annual trip, I was shocked to have my teacher Shastriji put a tourniquet on my left arm and shout a mantra at my third eye for five straight minutes. He said he was going to unravel my mind completely. Then I went to Madrid to rest, and I was flat out again for five straight days; I could not move. This time I was not going mad, but I could not move. I prayed constantly. Help came at last. A healer from Majorca walked in the door. While she worked on my body for three hours, kneading it like bread dough, she saw many past lives. Then she said I was going to have to go through the resurrection.

I was scheduled to go to San Sebastian, but I could not get on the plane without help. My assistant that week was a wealthy Chinese millionaire. (I remember she was wearing Armani clothes in the Madrid airport.) At the presentation, one hundred people were waiting for me. I could hardly stand up, and I was soaking wet again. I decided I was going on stage no matter what. I started sharing in Spanish what was happening to me. Then suddenly I *was* resurrected, and right in front of them. A frightfully loud sound roared through the electrical system as if it had its own kundalini coming toward me. When that blast came out of the microphone, it had such a force that it entered my body, and I jumped right in front of everyone. I was healed! I was resurrected right then and there. I still wonder what those people thought. Anyway, the Spanish people always love me, always accept me.

I spent the year recovering from that initiation. But that year in India, Shastriji put tourniquets on both my arms and shouted mantras again. I had this treatment three times. I should have known the next year might be even harder. *Harder?* What an understatement! My final initiation was the hardest thing in my whole life.

Initiation into the Void

It was December 1, 1994, eleven days before the important evolutionary leap called 12:12. On this day, vibrations were altered on the earth, new amino acids were triggered in our bodies with new hydrogen matrices, and a spiritual quickening happened, making aging and death optional. I should have known something major would happen to me. Look what happened to me on 11:11! But I went ahead with my plans to go to Egypt to join others who were going there for more knowledge on Physical Immortality. Because I had been there before and had taken a tour, I agreed this time to be a leader on one of the boats. Many other leaders were going, fortunately, because I did not make it.

On December 1, I was standing before my colleague's lovely altar in Santa Fe, enjoying the essence of Quan Yin. I felt totally innocent. Suddenly, a force from outside my body hit me very hard over the heart area. At the same moment, the woman of the house came down for our meeting, so I did not mention it. I thought it was unusual all right, but we continued with our meeting, and I thought the effect would go away. After that meeting, I was knocked out flat at Emily Goldman's house, where I was always cared for. I could not move, but the next day I was in the car, going to the airport anyway. I began shaking quite violently, and Emily's daughter Victoria informed me she was not taking me to the airport. I said, "Oh, this is just some kundalini moving. I will be all right." But I was not all right. I could not get on the plane. I thought, "Oh, I will just go tomorrow instead." But the next day was worse. I was in a thoroughly strange state. That night I received a call from a guide in Puerto Rico. She said, "A man wearing white robes has appeared with flowers for you; he is laying them at your feet and saying you

145

are not to go to Egypt. You are to stay where you are and have your own private initiation in seclusion." I had to resign myself to the fact that I was not going to Egypt. But that was not the main problem. The main problem was that I felt like someone had grabbed my heart area and was squeezing it. The pain was almost intolerable.

I called my friend and confessed to her what had happened at her home. She said maybe I had been hit with energies from the Middle East that were flying around her house—or dark forces. I did not like that reply at all. I did not want to believe in dark forces and make them real. She said, "Well, call it the cosmic ego." That thought only frightened me. Were forces trying to stop me? I became utterly paranoid. A multitude of turbulent past lives came up in which I had been assassinated for being ahead of my time—assassinated by groups of people who had harassed me for years. The past lives were absolutely terrifying to remember. I laid by the fire and a heavy, overpowering energy surrounded me. I became more paranoid. I felt that people were out to get me. Never in my life had I been a fearful person. I was not used to feeling fear, and I could not imagine where all the fear came from.

That was all occurring at the same time that my whole organization was completely ripped apart. I had no support from people on my staff except for one or two dedicated members. Everyone seemed to enter into some horrendous past life we had together. Everything was weird, dark, and torn apart. I could not tell which life I was in, who was supporting me, and who was not. I felt I could not trust anyone. I was alone and felt totally unsupported—except that Emily and Victoria, who had been at ashrams with me many times, were there for me. Diana also called me every day. Their concern kept me sane. I could not eat. I was constantly terrified . . . of what, I did not know.

I called Beth for help. She came over and sat with me, and all she told me was that for two years, one of my teachers had prepared me for this. It was an "initiation into the void." She said I must go through it alone. She added that I was to open my heart to the level that Gandhi had attained, and that was going to be difficult—that I must learn to feel compassion for the whole world. I was given no more information. I felt desperate. I could not clear my body; nothing worked. None of the old techniques were right for this process. I did not understand the oppressive energy at all. Emily would build a fire, and I would lie by the fireplace and listen to the Aarti, which helped somewhat. Another thing that helped was Rolfing. My Rolfer came and gave me three sessions that week. That made me feel saner. She was extremely supportive.

Sometimes I got too much fear in my body, and I would actually go and get in Emily's bed. She was very kind that way and very stable, and she would just get up and be with me during the night. None of us slept much. Something had taken over. It was impossible to figure out. I began calling some clairvoyants for help. I needed help. I felt desperate for help, actually. People were very kind to me, but nobody could really explain what was happening. I was able to get help clearing the past lives coming up. But that was only one aspect of the whole process. I cried almost continuously. If I could not have cried, I would have gone crazy. I wrote to my gurus and put the letters on the altar. One wrote me back and told me to *shake out* the fear—and that was all. Obviously, I was not to have much information. I had to learn to *trust* more, and that was not easy when I felt terrible. But at least I was not sick.

Finally, on December 11, I felt they had had enough, and I needed to give everyone in that house a break. I got on a plane, went to Los Angeles, and stayed with old friends. But I was still a mess. I either had a severe gripping feeling over my heart chakra or I had terror going up and down my spine. I had to stay very close to my friends who were breathworkers. One day I made a decision to go to the Jose Eber salon in Beverly Hills for a complete makeover. During this period, my old friend Bobby Birdsall took care of me. At the salon, he watched all the gorgeous women while I had a makeover. I figured that I was changing completely, so why not a new hairdo? These little things helped. I hung around the old-timers, such as Mannie and Annie, who were fun. I needed *fun*— simple things to keep me in my body. During this time, I could not work. I was running out of money. I had to cancel several events, including a conference in Israel. No way could I have handled Israel in that state. Being in such a condition is the worst nightmare for a performer or public figure.

But there were a few things I could not cancel. Before Christmas, I had to go to Salt Lake City to conduct an event and then attend an evening event in Portland. In Salt Lake, I had a difficult time on stage, which is unusual for me. It felt as though glass was shattering in my spine, and I felt like I would faint. But nobody knew and I was able to finish the event. When I got to Portland, I decided to sit down for the whole presentation. Fortunately, the universe agreed and provided a couch for me on the stage. I was in a church. I told the people that I must do my devotions in public with them, because I was going through too much. That was the right decision.

During the Divine Mother prayers, I saw a lovely blonde woman in the audience having a "religious experience." She was shaking and crying. I hoped that she would come and tell me about it at the break and she did. She stood in line to speak to me; then she shared that she had seen my guru Babaji on stage with me.

"Thank God," I said, "I need to know if he said anything." She told me he had said that *I had now become the cave and he is taking off the trousers.* I understood his message at some level; but I asked her to come and sit with me at the end of the presentation, which she did. I *wanted* to be like the cave, the womb of the Divine Mother in Herakhan, where my guru had materialized his body. This meant I was becoming what I needed to become. And "taking off the trousers" meant, I assumed, that he was getting me out of the masculine side of my being to the feminine side, where I belonged. For years, I had to be the masculine side, on the "front lines" in the patriarchal energy. Had I not, I would have been quite sick. Now was the right time, and it was safe enough for me to switch. This switch was one of the most difficult ordeals in my life as a public figure. I had to change at the deepest level. I had to confront every one of my fears of being a female leader. Being a male leader was easier. I had done it numerous times before.

At the end, she and her mother came and sat with me. The mother had the same name as me: *Sondra.* How symbolic! It was amazing. I sat across from Sondra, who just loved me, while the daughter, Oshara, a pure clairvoyant, told me the following: "There is a being behind you who is like an alien, very tall, and he is holding a long, long scroll of names of women who had made an 'agreement' to allow the patriarchy to take over."

"Obviously to balance the karma of the matriarchy," I thought.

She said that he was telling me I must be the one to break this pact. I must decide if I was willing to take this responsibility. Then he disappeared and she told me I would have to face him later. I took this as another test to see if I was, after all I had endured, still willing to take the responsibility for the Divine Mother movement.

I returned to Los Angeles. In the home of Dana and Peter, "the being" confronted me again. He appeared to me one night. He was tall and his ears were different from human ears. I stood up to him and agreed. I woke up in a cold sweat, terrified again. These experiences were over my head. I had to call Ashanna for help. She kept telling me I was stronger than my fear, which was the right thing to say.

At night, I began to see new blueprints actually entering my body. It was all code to me, and I did not understand it at all. In one dream, I saw my own kundalini lying on the floor. I picked it up and ran through the halls of a university looking for someone to explain to me what was happening. I was told that a professor at the end of the hall knew everything. A very long line was waiting for him. When I reached him, I said, "I only need five minutes of your time." He said, "You can have ten." But then I woke up and did not get the answer from him.

This was absolutely a process for me to go through alone. I had to get my own answers—and they were not coming fast enough to satisfy me. I had to surrender and trust. It was so humbling, this experience, because I could not figure it out at all. Nor were the answers in any book. I was shocked it went on so long. I grew discouraged and I had to continually choose to live. I remember thinking that I was having a nervous breakdown, but that did not turn out to be true at all. It was the death of my ego, and it was a constant battle.

Then I had to go to Japan. "I am too fragile," I thought; so I asked Diana to go with me, thank God. We were there shortly after the earthquake and one week before the gassings in the underground subways. I went a week early to acclimate. I had tremendous resistance to Japan. The little apartments made me feel as though I were in a box all the time. Then there was a another major earthquake warning, the very day I was to teach Physical Immortality to the Japanese. I felt that was my real test. Had I become strong enough to face *that* without going nuts? I told Diana we should take the bull by the horns and move right into the heart of Tokyo and start chanting. I called up two Japanese devotees of Babaji and invited them over to our hotel room, also a little box. (Diana said, "We are moving from one box to another.") I felt that the earthquake actually could happen, because people still had so much fear from the last one that they could have easily re-created another. Also, this one was predicted by a little boy who had super powers, and he had accurately predicted the first. I thought it might occur around three o'clock in the morning before my class. At that time, on the button, my organizers were in a taxi that was hit from behind and in front at the same time—and their heads were knocked together. They came to the class in shock. I went ahead and started teaching, not knowing if the earthquake might still come that day.

I got a different kind of earthquake. A lovely man from Canada showed up to that seminar, and we had a very strong connection. (As it turned out, there actually was an earthquake, but it was under the sea.)

Fortunately for me, I was going to Maui for the next stop on my tour. On the day I reached Maui, glass shattered around me on three occasions, while all the tensions of Japan came out of my body. Maui healed me tremendously. The last night after my advanced seminar of Physical Immortality, I was lying around with the assistants. Then it did happen: a minor earthquake occurred then and there. The couch was vibrating and undulating. Actually, it was quite sensual. I started feeling I was going to make it.

And now I had to go back to work seriously. I had a long European tour ahead. But more terrifying past lives continued to come up. I had hoped I was finished—but no such luck. In Poland, I had a kind of accident when I slammed the bathroom door in someone's house: a bracket came right off the door and sent me flying across the room. I landed upside down in the bathtub (with my clothes on). Then I had to return to the training session I was conducting at the time, very shaken and in pain. Fortunately, I had scheduled that past-life session in the home of four doctors. I did not need them, however, except for homeopathy for shock. That was a fairly rough training session because my cotrainer started vomiting after the birth section, and my translator had diarrhea and had to run off the stage. The Polish people, however, were just wonderful. I experienced the power of Poland . . . and never have I seen so much gratitude.

In Spain, I had the miracle of being able to see Jose again. He seemed totally aware of what I was going through, as usual; and he was the first one who could adequately explain things to me. He told me that new channels had opened up in me for later work. It was very important, and I had to be willing to "sacrifice for God." He told me that he, too, ended up on the floor many times, unable to work because of the changes he had to go through. I felt better after that. He helped me integrate the energy. He renewed my confidence that all was in order.

I then took a pilgrimage to the remote site of the Virgin in Garabalde, Spain, for Holy Thursday before Easter. I felt I should fast and do penance. It was a long train ride, a long bus ride, and after that, a hike uphill. I asked several people to go with me, but they could not. Again, I had to do it alone. But after all, I had been to Medjurorje, Yugoslavia, alone. I was still fragile, but I knew this would give me strength. Also, Jose had told me I would receive a "gift."

I was in shock to find out what it is like to travel in Spain on trains during Easter. The train station was packed—like in India, body to body. I had gotten the last spot. After eight hours on the train, I changed to a bus and began the long bus ride on very curvy roads high up in the mountains. Behind me sat a woman who carried on a conversation the entire time (two and a half hours) with someone who was not there. She constantly chatted to this person next to her, but I did not see anyone in that seat. Across from me was a priest from somewhere. He kept yelling at his assistant, and his assistant kept yelling at him. The priest was really loud mouthed and terribly cranky. And yet, when we stopped in a café for coffee, people treated him as though he were God—"Father this" and Father that," and a stranger paid for his food. He remained cranky the whole time.

When we got to the site I thought was a village, I was surprised to find that it was a mountain we must climb. I had the wrong shoes for that and a bag that was far too heavy. I felt very critical of myself for this lack of common sense. But I reminded myself that I had been though very stressful times, I was fortunate not to be sick, and I could forgive myself for mistakes like this. Then approaching me was a little man in a pinstriped suit from the 1930s that had never been dry-cleaned, if you ask me. He was terribly sweet and offered to help carry my bag. We made a funny team, him carrying one handle and me the other, since we were so different in size. I asked him if we had to climb to the top of the mountain, hoping that the

site was a bit lower. He said, "Of course, madam." I finally found a
tienda where I could leave my bag, and I actually found some ten-
nis shoes to buy in the little village we passed. Of course, they did
not really fit.

At the top, I stayed for quite a few hours at the site where the
Virgin had materialized. I lay on the grass with everyone else in that
precious energy. It was bliss, really.

When it came time for me to hike down, I had a real shock.
Crowds of people were climbing up and really struggling with their
breathing and fatigue, leaning on their canes or the stronger arm of
another person. I saw one woman coming up carrying a huge baby.
When she got closer, I realized she was not carrying a baby at all.
She was carrying a man, only he had no arms and no legs. I wept to
think of his tragic state and her loving compassion. I still cannot
stop thinking about it.

Later in the chapel during the mass, more new energy entered
my body while the priests performed the traditional washing of the
feet of twelve men. I was very glad I had come. But the problem was
that I had to leave before the bus came so I could make it back to a
train that would get me back to Madrid in time. After all, a man was
flying in to see me, and I wanted to see him. I decided I would
hitchhike if necessary.

As it turned out, I saw a man sitting alone in a nice car. I asked
him if he was, by chance, going back to Santander. He said, "Yes," as
if he were just waiting for me. Strange. He drove me to Santander
in his nice car, playing nice music on the stereo all the way. The next
day the man I had been seeing for a couple of years came to Madrid.
I needed this break. By some mysterious coincidence, he had just
returned from Fatima in Portugal.

On this trip, I also had the great privilege of meeting Mother
Meera, the Indian avatar, living in a small village in Germany. I had
waited years for the opportunity, and that was the right time. We
had to sit three hours in absolute silence while she worked on us
one by one, helping to remove obstacles. Thousands of people
come from all over the world to have her *darshan.* I had been told
she was one of my main guides for the Divine Mother movement,
along with Mother Mary, so I felt it was important to go at this
time. The unique gift she brings is to make available the transfor-
mative Light of Paramatman, the Supreme Being. She offers a

direct transmission of this Light, and obviously, she is like a transformer, reducing it down for us to be able to tolerate it. I would recommend her book *Answers*.

Because of these wonderful experiences with the Divine Mother, I was able to go on and handle some very tough assignments alone. Before, I always had cotrainers, assistants, or bodyworkers with me. This time I had to do everything alone. Even in Italy, when a blind student had an epileptic seizure during a session, I had to handle it alone; my organizers were out of the room at the time. After I got everyone centered, the assistants and students came forth to help. But basically, the tragic crisis required my strength to calm everyone. The fear in the room was intense. I had been through so much fear already that I became remarkably calm, although I continued to experience one test after another.

However, when I got to London, Diana had to do breathwork on me off and on for three days. I also needed acupuncture, chiropractic, and Rolfing. I was burned out. But when I got to the evening of my speech, I experienced such a power roaring through me that there was nothing I had ever felt to which I could compare it. I was different, so different that I got on a plane and flew to Majorca. In two days, I found a darling chalet near a lovely beach that I decided to rent for a year. I was beginning my new life.

PART VI

Conclusions

The Last Initiation

I was determined to heal myself completely and permanently and I even wanted transfiguration of my body. After all, Jesus said, "All things are possible," didn't he? *A Course in Miracles* says the healing of God's Son is all the world is for so I took that to mean, quite literally, that I was here to get healed and totally liberated. It was all going fairly well for me until my mother died. On the first anniversary of her death, I hit a wall. I landed in Germany to work, and suddenly I was unable to digest food. This also had happened to me after my sister's death, but this time it was much worse. I had severe pain if I ate. The situation became very grave. Then the unthinkable happened. It got so bad I had to quit work. I no longer had the sparkling energy with which I helped others to heal themselves. I felt quite literally dead and I became so thin that my friends checked me into a hospital. My insurance would not cover "anorexia" so I soon lost all my inheritance.

I finally hit rock bottom and entered the Dark Night of the Soul.

Having no siblings or parents left flipped me into a deep depression that was exacerbated by lack of nutrition and vice versa.

The following three years were my hardest test of all. I could not work and I was a basket case after twenty-seven years of traveling. I was burned out and I could not go on. I finally ended up in a spiritual community started by Jessica Dibb in Baltimore where they "took me in." I went into seclusion living with a woman named Pat who was like a yogi. I almost never came out of my room. Now I can say I finally understand why yogis go into caves. I call those three years my "Cave Period." Some would call it the Dark Night of the Soul. Caroline Myss, the great medical intuitive, calls it "spiritual madness." She obviously must have gone through it because she was able to describe it better than anyone. Fortunately someone sent me her tape so I had some idea what was going on with me.

When you are severely depressed, it is obviously due to the death urge coming out. I knew all that, but I had no motivation for the first time in my life, and that was harder for me to get out of than any of the physical diseases I mention in this book. However, I can now say that this experience was the most profound thing in my life.

And I *finally* was able to resurrect myself.

Carolyn says that after you invoke very direct contact with God, everything eventually gets turned upside down. Your whole life gets reordered and every false voice is taken away.

She said that you get separated from the world you knew and you experience a breakdown in the human order. All distractions are taken away and you go into yourself alone and face your shadow side. Thoughts of suicide even come and you enter the tomb and go through the Lazarus experience. That is exactly what happened to me.

For me it felt like hell. I truly began to understand why *A Course in Miracles* said, "Hell is what the ego makes of the present." I was creating my own hell and I knew it. Biblical characters called it the "pit" or the "belly of the whale." Jessica kept telling me one saint was in it for twelve years. I did not want to face *that*. I had no money to rely on my usual healers. I would have to get out of this one myself. I really could not let in much support, but those people protected me.

I had done a lot of work on my personal shadow with breath-work, but I had not completed the "family shadow" and the "religious shadow." For months and months I was dealing with the family mind over and over and over. I even got in touch with the genetics of my ancestors. Then I was dealing with religious guilt day in and day out. I felt so guilty I could not even open the spiritual books that I knew would help me. I was too guilty. So many past lives came up that I could hardly shake them off. Once a week I would drag myself out of bed, force myself to walk to Jessica's, and let her do breathwork on me. It was even hard to get much breath going. But she somehow kept me going. I just did not see the point of living if I could not work and make a contribution and my whole family was gone. I had no desire to see anyone. Pat, who had been through cancer, just let me be and was completely nonjudgmental and looked after me for a year with unconditional love.

I finally got the nerve to call a medical sensitive on the East Coast. I could not afford many calls to her but one was enough. She told me flat out that I was going to have to get off the fence. I knew what she meant. I had very little will to live and I had to choose. Only it is hard to choose when you are so depressed.

It was getting close to New Year's Day, 2000. That was the day I consciously made the decision to force myself to give it a try and start doing spiritual practices again. I made a deal with my guru. I would do my part. Of course, God does help those who help themselves. I took advantage of all the universal energy being put out New Year's Eve right before the New Millennium.

The next day I began reading *A Course in Miracles* again, doing prayers, doing mantras and doing processes, and walking Pat's dog, Bodhi. I actually did approximately six to eight hours of spiritual practice a day for nine months. The ninth month Rhonda and Jeff got me out of there and took me to Venezuela to work. I was very shaky, but at least I was moving.

Later after it was all over, I finally understood what Caroline Myss said: "One has to make a commitment to explore the states on a downward spiral with the intention to experience them fully . . . like a deliberate descent into an inner Hell with the intention to clear one's system. Before the ego can be let go of, it must be known and understood in all its extremes." My Higher Self had chosen this experience and somehow I knew that because I had told my guru I wanted all that he had to offer.

I found out that what looked like madness to my peers—who knew the shape I was in—was really my true liberation. I had to rise above the shame that people thought I would never recover. The ego was coming out. This became more important to me than what people were saying about me. I saw the insanity of it all pass by. I understood why *A Course in Miracles* says the ego is insane. The hardest part for me was clearing family genetics. At one point I went through my grandfather's mind. He had had a chemical imbalance of the brain. This I more or less knew about, but I really found out it was true because I went through it myself. Now I am convinced one can get through *anything*. But if you give up, you will get stuck. During one part I had pain in my knees for six months. Everyone told me I had arthritis. If I had bought into that, I would have it now. I finally figured out it was just fear. When I forced myself to go back to work, it left.

Carolyn says most people choose *not* to have this experience. It is really for Initiated Souls who can handle the deepest and the darkest. I was more than lucky that I had chosen to be initiated by Babaji. By his grace, I am feeling wonderful now. I knew I had the "choice." I could check out and die and have to reincarnate and have to go through another birth trauma and another set of parents and yet another life of dogma from school, or I could keep on processing this out. I decided it was a small price to pay for Liberation. That was what I really wanted. If I didn't do it now, I would just have to do it all again in another life.

I was forced to live in the simplest manner with next to nothing. There was something very powerful about having to choose to live with nothing external to attract me. I had no money left for healers and treats or shopping. It was all just me and God. By the grace of Babaji, I made it. One night in a dream, I entered a library. It was all white. The walls were white, the shelves were white, the books were white, and Babaji appeared wearing all white. He took a book off the shelf and opened it up for me to see. He showed me a white brain that was regenerating. He taught me literally that anything can be healed by God. I clung to the verse, "There is nothing the Holy Spirit cannot handle by offering me a miracle."

Because of all my spiritual work over the years and because of my connection with the masters, which I had cultivated, I was taken care of by the universe in miraculous ways, too numerous to mention. At one point I got back to California, thanks to my friend Rhonda. I remained hidden in a center in an obscure area. The night it really started to turn around is when Natalie, a Babaji devotee, drove me to see Ammachi, my female guru, who happened to be visiting Los Angeles. It was like all the work I had done to serve the Divine Mother suddenly took hold. She held me in her arms and I remembered why I was here and my depression lifted!

I began to go to a simple Catholic church and pray to the Virgin. I was never Catholic but I liked the fact that this church was always open. I was staying in a simple Spanish neighborhood by the airport. I wondered what I was doing there. I did lots and lots of mantras day and night. When September 11 happened, I realized it was good I was there to do mantras and maybe Babaji had planned that. I did more and more mantras and more and more prayers. Finally I realized it was time to come out and work again in public. I began doing free spiritual events of chanting to help ward off terrorism. After all the Keys of Enosh says: "And when the people of God are assembled, their collective efforts will become so powerful that their prayers and mantras used collectively actually offset wars and terrorist activity."

I knew the Divine Mother wanted me to do this and when I started these free evenings, miracles began to happen again and my faith was restored.

The best thing was that I got over my writer's block. This block had tormented me for three years. It took a miracle to get me over writer's block and it happened this way. One of the neighbors saw me frequently go out and use the pay phone in front of his shop. He apparently kept asking his neighbor, "Who *is she?*" He could not figure me out and it bothered him because he was a clairvoyant. I did not look like I belonged in that neighborhood and he also thought I was like a Rubik's Cube! Finally he came out and we met. I gave him a picture of my guru Babaji and asked him if he got any messages. He said yes immediately. I hesitated. I was afraid Babaji might be mad at me for being so behind in my projects. I told him I was not ready for two days. I prepared myself and went back in two days, shaking. Babaji came through so loving, but then about the book he said there were too many "delays." That was the kick in the butt I needed. The next day I started writing. It was a miracle. Carlos, my Brazilian neighbor, saved the day.

One day I even wrote a new training called The Next Level. I had been released from my old obsolete belief systems. I had been healed of my self-inflicted separation from my Holy Christ Self, I had ascended out of my distorted pain-racked body and I had leaped into a new dimension. Out of sheer gratitude I felt impelled to share the spiritual practices that had gotten me out of the "belly of the whale." I was now experiencing a gradual restoration and rejuvenation of my body!

I once again felt the intent of wanting to be the most powerful force of good that I was capable of being. I forgave myself for my former self-aggrandizement of my ego and all my mistakes and I experienced the joy of my own personal transfiguration.

About this time I began intense prayers of gratitude, especially to the Divine Mother (the Intelligence behind Matter). After all, I *finally* figured out the secret of all my gurus. They prayed night and day to the Divine Mother. Babaji, in fact, had said as his departing words when he took conscious Samadhi, "I leave everything in the hands of the Divine Mother." I remembered I had dedicated myself to the mission of the Divine Mother Movement and it was phenomenal to be back on purpose after three long years of purification.

I share here a prayer I began reading out loud to the Divine Mother.

> *Praise to you, Divine Mother, you have once again made my life a miracle. I take refuge in your nurturing arms of compassion. I praise you for once again giving me a spirit of power and love and sound mind. I praise all you have created and I want your name to be exalted. You called me out of darkness to your marvelous light. I shout with the voice of triumph. I offer myself willingly to you. Great and marvelous are your works. May all nations worship before you. I fall down before you and worship you who lives forever and ever. I praise you for your excellent greatness. With you all things are possible. I am humbled and bowed down as you are revealed to me. You have destroyed the last enemy in me and made me alive once again. You have raised me from the dust and from the ash heap. I sing praises to your powers because you have revived my heart. You brought me back to life, therefore I glorify you in my spirit and body. Let me declare your glory among the nations. I want to always obey your voice and be your treasure on this land. You have removed the burden from my shoulders. As your servant, I will do your will from my heart. If you will a thing for me to do, I will do it as perfectly as I can and give the glory to you. Let us all praise your name and greatness.*
>
> *As a newborn baby, I desire the milk of your word. I have been born again and I love you as a heir to your Kingdom. Thank you for accepting my repentance and giving me victory. You are my salvation. In you, Mother,*

I have peace. You have delivered me and put a new song in my mouth. I will serve you with gladness. I am lying at your divine feet and feeling pleased with the grace of your protection. You are the embodiment of Ultimate Bliss. You are supreme.

You have crowned my life with success and liberation. You are the essence of all that can be known. You are beyond comprehension. You have taken the form of my supreme Guru Babaji by whose grace I have been allowed to live again. The love of your lotus feet gives me lasting happiness. Glory to You, oh Mother of the Universe.

Everything I do is a result of your Divine Energy moving through me. I wish to express my appreciation to you as the source of all life. You are the breath of life. I am simply your instrument. You are my only goal in life. I desire that all should worship you Day and Night.

I offer up my song to nobody else but you.

I offer up my heart to nobody else but you.

My heart cries out for more of you.

My soul cries out for more of you.

My life is under your command.

I ask you to guide and assist me in fulfilling the mission I volunteered to do on Earth prior to this embodiment. I open myself completely to you so that I can manifest what I vowed to accomplish during this incarnation. I agree to be part of cocreating the new world with you to the best of my ability. What shall we do and how shall we do it? Show us the way.

Ignite us all with illumination.

On finding you, everything is found. You are the instrument of the Healing of the world.

Oh that all of our actions be that of worship, our words like Hymns. May your knowledge triumph. Teach us all the language of your heart. I believe you will guide us. Oh call on me. Show me what to write and say. Let the words of my mouth be acceptable to you. How can I convince mankind that you are the answer? I will tell the whole world of your irresistible miracles in my next book and I pray that everyone will see that nothing is too hard for you. It is you who can destroy the pain of this world. It is due to you that we will be able to release our sorrows. It is due to you that we shall find true happiness.

Show us the way.

To You I give all the Glory.

Love, Sondra Ray!

Sacred Renewal™ Breathwork

During these crucial times ahead, everything must be taken to the next level where new paradigms are needed. This also applies to the breathwork. We have done great work in the past decades; however, now we need to work with the highest vibration possible.

The great saint, Sri Auorobindo, said that the final stage of perfection is surrender to the Divine Mother. In India, they say that there is nothing higher than worship of the Divine Mother. The Divine Mother vibration needs to be emphasized now like never before, since we can see by our results in the world how out of balance we actually are. The sacred feminine has been so suppressed for so long that we have lost touch with our true essence. In each of us there is a masculine side and a feminine side. We are all so out of balance that we are addicted to the masculine side and chauvinism runs rampant. Men and women both have been taught to equate masculinity with domination and violence. This problem is accentuated by many religious dogmas. The model of the universe in which a male God rules the cosmos serves to legitimize male control in social institutions. But systems cannot merely be rejected when they aren't working; they must be replaced. Nor would it work to replace the system with the Matriarchy.

However, historically peace came where the Divine Mother was worshipped by both men and women, who ruled together as equals. No one dominated anyone. When we speak of the Divine Mother, we are referring to the original spark of creation, which is a feminine aspect. The Prime Creator behind all things is a female vibration. The Divine Mother is the Feminine aspect of God, or better said to be the "intelligence behind matter." Einstein knew this. All my male gurus in India who I admire so much know this. It is the very secret of their power. We are talking about true power here: love, safety, and certainty, not ego power, which is domination, control, and anger.

When people surrender to the Divine Mother, extraordinary changes take place. When you explore the Goddess energy you truly value life. The Divine Mother is the Source of all knowledge, beyond everything, and the true release from delusion. This essence of the life force (shakti) cannot be controlled. The Divine Mother as kundalini will clean you out. Your old personality becomes replaced by miracle consciousness. The greater your devotion to her, the faster your progress. It is due to her we can achieve true happiness. It is due to her transcendent nature and personification of intelligence that matter is created. Everything we possess is a gift from the Mother. When we surrender to her, the intelligence of the whole universe is our teacher. We have the urge to bring forth the inexpressible into manifestation. We remember the ecstasy of being alive! Our bodies can become instruments through which the feminine aspect plays.

Men need to learn to be more sensitive and intuitive and women need to learn to thrive in their own power. Are you, for example, a woman who grew up pleasing rather than being? And do you do almost anything to avoid a man's irritation? Did you immerse yourself in the values of a male-dominated society? Did you reorder your priorities and give your power away just to please a man? Wouldn't you rather be a fully awakened woman with a balanced feminine and masculine side? The more balanced you are, the deeper your relationships can be with all human beings.

Are you a man who is afraid to feel his feelings, afraid to show softness and tenderness? Do you feel pressure to becoming a money-producing machine? Are you afraid to give up your anger for fear of becoming weak?

Wouldn't you rather become a fully awakened male who is in balance, who could easily channel the right solutions for the world and provide the right environment for physical, emotional, mental, and spiritual progress?

What if tapping into the Divine Mother energy in a balanced way to produce regeneration, restoration, and renewal? The Divine Mother has shown me her renewal abilities in miraculous ways. I have the great honor to be writing about that for my next book.

I also have the great honor to spread the Divine Mother Movement in the world to help balance our civilization. And so the Divine Mother has asked me to take the breathwork we have been doing to the next level. She asked me to use the words "Sacred Renewal" for the new paradigm in this healing modality. The breathworkers who choose to be part of this new work will be preparing for sessions in a new way. They will be doing deep prayers given to me by my gurus before each session. They will be doing mantras during the session. They will be using sound therapy for putting the brain in sync at the end of the session; and the sessions will be done in healing temples. I am so thrilled that the sacredness of this work will be emphasized. So far in my experiments the results are much deeper, smoother, safer, softer, more beneficial, more ecstatic, and more regenerative. Each renewal session is dedicated by the guide to the Divine Mother, the complete healing of the person and the healing of the earth. The breathworker will be required to go through a special initiation guided by my male and female masters.

My prayer is that everyone who needs healing of any kind, can experience the benefits of this renewal work.

It is no mistake that I wrote this just after seeing my female Divine Mother teachers, Karunamayi and Ammachi. To them, with great devotion, I say, "Oh teach me to surrender to you totally so that we can move forward with this work."

To you, the reader:

If you would like Sondra Ray to speak in your community, your workplace, or at any public event or conference, visit the website www.SondraRay.com or call 888-800-5034.

If you would like Sondra and Sharda to train your meditation group, prayer group, *A Course in Miracles* study group, club, or any other group on how to do Sacred Renewal™ Breathwork on each other, please see the website www.SondraRay.com or call toll free in the U.S. 888-800-5034.

If you are interested in traveling with Sondra and Sharda on the following spiritual trips, please call 727-363-6685.

- Travel to India and deepen your connection to the Divine Mother.

- Travel to Bali to visit sacred sites and to enhance your physical immortality.

- Or other future spiritual trips.

Thank you for telling others about this book. *A Course in Miracles* says, "Nothing real can be increased except by sharing."

I am looking forward to meeting you soon.

Sondra Ray!

Bibliography

Airola, Paavo. *Are You Confused? The Authoritative Answers to Controversial Questions.* Health Plus Publishing, 1971.

Amriteswarupananda, Swami. *Awaken Children.* M.A. Center.

Busch, Heather, and Burton Silver. *Why Cats Paint: A Theory of Feline Aesthetics.* Berkeley, Calif.: Ten Speed Press, 1994.

Chopra, Deepak. *Quantum Healing: Exploring the Frontiers of Mind Body Medicine.* New York: Bantam, 1990.

_____. *Unconditional Life: Discovering the Power to Fulfill Your Dreams.* New York: Bantam, 1992.

Dalai Lama. "A Human Approach to World Peace."

Essene, Virgina, ed. *New Cells, New Bodies, New Life! You're Becoming a Fountain of Youth!* Santa Clara, Calif.: S.E.E. Publishing Co., 1991.

Ferguson, Marilyn. "The Paradigm of Proven Potentials." *New Sense Bulletins*

Ferrini, Paul. *Love Without Conditions: Reflections of the Christ Mind.* Greenfield, Mass.: Heartways Press, 1994.

Foundation for Inner Peace. *A Course in Miracles.* Foundation for Inner Peace, 1975.

Goodman, Linda. *Linda Goodman's Star Signs.* New York: St Martin's Press, 1987.

Hay, Louise L. *Heal Your Body: The Mental Causes for Physical Illness and the Metaphysical Way to Overcome Them.* Carlsbad, Calif.: Hay House, 1994.

Johnson, Robert A. *Transformation: Understanding the Three Levels of Masculine Consciousness.* New York: HarperCollins, 1991.

Leibman, Joshua. *Peace of Mind.* New York: Citadel Press, 1994.

Meera, Mother. Meeramma Publications.

Muktananda, Swami. *Play of Consciousness: A Spiritual Autobiography.* New York: Syda Foundation, 1994.

Ponder, Catherine. *The Dynamic Laws of Healing.* Marina del Rey, Calif.: Devorss and Co., 1989.

Ray, Sondra. *Essays on Creating Sacred Relationships—The Next Step to a New Paradigm.* Berkeley, Calif.: Celestial Arts, 1996.

_____. *How to Be Chic, Fabulous, and Live Forever.* Berkeley, Calif.: Celestial Arts, 1992.

_____. *Loving Relationships II: The Secrets of a Great Relationship.* Berkeley, Calif.: Celestial Arts, 1990.

_____. *The Only Diet There Is.* Berkeley, Calif.: Celestial Arts, 1982.

_____. *Pur Joy.* Berkeley, Calif.: Celestial Arts, 1988.

_____. *Rebirthing in the New Age.* Berkeley, Calif.: Celestial Arts, 1993

Robbins, John. *Diet for a New America: How Your Food Choices Affect Your Health, Happiness, and the Future of Life on Earth.* Novato, Calif.: H.J. Kramer, 1998.

Roberts, Jane. *The Nature of the Psyche: Its Human Expression.* A Seth Book. San Rafael, Calif.: Amber-Allen Publishing, 1996.

Svoboda, Robert E. *Aghora: At the Left Hand of God and the Kundalini* series. Las Vegas, Nev.: Brotherhood of Life, 1986.

Tannen, Deborah. *You Just Don't Understand.* New York: Quill, 2001.

Watson, Lyall. *The Romeo Error: A Matter of Life and Death.* New York: Doubleday, 1975.

Williamson, Marianne. *Return to Love: Reflections on the Principles of a Course in Miracles.* New York: HarperCollins, 1996.

Woolger, Roger J. *Other Lives, Other Selves: A Jungian Psychotherapist Discovers Past Lives.* New York: Bantam Books, 1988.

World Ascension Network Newsletters.

Yogananda, Paramahansa. *Autobiography of a Yogi.* Nevada City, Calif.: Crystal Clarity Publishing, 1997.